Eat It Later

*Mastering Self Control &
The Slimming Power Of
Postponement*

By Michael Alvear

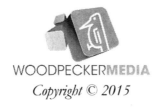

WOODPECKERMEDIA

Copyright © 2015

Table Of Contents

Introduction

If Oreos are proof that God exists then I was a fervent believer. I'd eat mounds of them and never gain weight. Skinny all my life, I ate fat and sugar bombs with impunity, earning admiration from many and ire from most. I was not familiar with the word "diet," though I had seen it on cans of Coke. It all came crashing down in my late 20s when I started to gain weight. The chickens had come home to roost and they weren't organic. They were vengeful. In short order I had gained 14 pounds and almost two pant sizes.

Suddenly I became intimately familiar with a truckload of diets and tried many variations of them, all to no avail. I found the idea of being on a diet the rest of my life, well, unappetizing. So I went on a quixotic quest for a way to lose weight without sacrificing my favorite foods.

This book is about how I lost 14 pounds and 2 waist sizes and kept it off for 25 years without ever going on a diet. Inspired by Walter Mischel's iconic The Marshmallow Test, I developed my own delayed gratification techniques, which painlessly—and dramatically—reduced the volume of food I ate. I then adapted strategies psychologists use to overcome drug addiction and phobias (systematic desensitization and habituation) and applied them to eating. The result? I stopped binging on problem foods.

Together, these strategies helped me do what few can: Eat

whatever I want in moderate portions. *Eat It Later* chronicles how I did it and lays out a plan for how readers can too. It's a 3-step process—*Reframe* your goals from weight loss to health enhancement, *Eliminate* binge eating through desensitization and *Reduce* the volume and frequency of problem food consumption through innovative delayed gratification techniques.

I wasn't overweight but I knew where I was headed when a friend said, *"You're two weeks away from being fat."* At 28 years old I noticed that my pants were getting tighter and tighter. I was angry at the dry cleaners—they were clearly using a process that shrunk my pants! I went from a size 32 waist to a size 34. At first, I just accepted it. After all, I was 6'1" and 175 lbs., hardly anyone's idea of fat. But it wasn't long before I was 185 lbs. And then not too long after that, 194 lbs.

Now, 6'1" and 194 lbs. is not fat but it's, well, two weeks away from it. Almost everybody who's been skinny or normal-weight all their life will face a moment of truth about their expanding middles. Mine came at Macy's. I tried on a pair of 34 waist pants. They were a little tight so I reached for a 36.

That's when the moment hit me. "If I try these on," I remember thinking, "I'm saying it's okay to keep gaining the weight. And if it's okay to go from 32 to 34 and then to 36 pretty soon it'll be okay to go from 36 to 38 and then where would it stop?"

I put the 36 pants back on the rack.

I knew if I didn't stop the weight gain right then and there, when it would be relatively easy to do it, I'd end up fat the rest of my life. I confronted the unthinkable: Skinny me, normal weight me, was about to get fat. I was in denial. "This happens to *other* people," I thought. "Not *me*." I pictured myself wobbling into restaurants that handed me estimates instead of menus. I even had a dream that I'd gotten so fat a cop told me that I could legally use the carpool lane, even when I travelled alone.

So I went on a quest to lose some weight. I went on every conceivable diet—Atkins, South Beach, Hollywood, low carb, high protein, and gluten free. You name it I tried it.

They all worked. But the suffering, the deprivation, the constant vigilance and oh, my God, the math, THE MATH! I had to count those calories, weigh these products, measure those foods, calcu-late the fat, subtract the salt, divide the carbs, move towards this, away from that, it was *exhausting.*

It's a 3-step process—
Reframe your goals from weight loss to health enhancement,
Eliminate binge eating through desensitization and
Reduce the volume and frequency of problem food consumption through innovative delayed gratification techniques.

Yes, I lost the weight but I was miserable and couldn't sustain it. I wanted to enjoy my food not feel victimized by it. I gained the weight right back and started scratching at the door of waist size 36.

Around that time I met a friend, Mike, an editor at a major health magazine. He vetted research on diet and weight loss. Mike completely changed the way I looked at dieting. For starters he introduced me to a body of research that showed what you no doubt already know: DIETS DON'T WORK. People almost always gain the weight back (present company included).

What fascinated me about the research Mike showed me was not just how unanimous it was about what *didn't* work, but about what did. And it was never about what foods to eat or avoid or which exercise regimen worked best. It was always about one thing and one thing only: Moderation. Portion control. Eating whatever you want but staying within the confines of reason.

There's only one problem: Moderation is often more difficult than dieting. It requires you to navigate the psychological obstacles to self-restraint, like managing urgent cravings, mastering the skill of delayed gratification, recognizing satiety, and dealing with wildly disruptive psychological phenomena that keep us from eating moderately, like the "DelBoeuf illusion" (plate size affects how much you eat).

According to Mike, the research was clear: The people who

could successfully manage these psychological obstacles lost weight *without having to go on a diet*. The successful people didn't have a food plan; they had an eating strategy.

Right. I looked at Mike the quizzical way an ostrich looks when it hears a whistle. I had no idea what he was talking about. "Come on, Mike," I said. "You're saying I just need to do a few Jedi mind tricks and I'd be able to eat nearly anything I want and lose weight?" It sounded like another empty diet book promise. But Mike was insistent. "First of all, he said, "They aren't Jedi mind tricks; they are eating strategies designed to neutralize recognized psychological roadblocks to weight loss."

He proposed a test. He knew I was an Oreo cookie addict. I'd eat 16 at a sitting. "I can get you to eat three using these principles," he said, "without you craving the other 13."

Right. "You're saying that I can go from eating 16 Oreos to 3 without experiencing withdrawals or overwhelming cravings for more?"

"Yes," he said. "And if I can prove that you can do it with Oreos—the thing you're most addicted to—imagine the success you'd have with cutting back other fattening foods."

Oh, it was on. I accepted the challenge. Mike sat me down and explained what would be involved. I followed his instructions to the letter and I was blown away by the results.

I went from eating 16 Oreos at a sitting to 3 without any cravings for more.

I was so shocked at my success I begged Mike to tell me about all the research he came across and I used the information to build a simple program to lose weight.

A program that didn't require me to count calories, carbs or proteins. A program that didn't require me to weigh my food or severely restrict my diet. A program that didn't require me to have anything but a rudimentary knowledge of which foods were healthy or unhealthy.

The result? I lost 14 pounds and two pant sizes.

I know what you're thinking: "Big deal! You can achieve that with any diet!" True, *but I wasn't on a diet.* That's the point. I lost fourteen pounds and almost two waist sizes by changing the way I ate, not what I ate. And the results have been permanent. I went from almost a size 36 waist to a comfortable size 32 and have been there for the past 25 years.

Twenty-five years!

And wait, it gets worse. I don't cook. I eat out nearly half to two thirds of my meals.

How did I do it? Through a series of psychological strategies that painlessly reduced urgent cravings, dramatically increased my ability to delay gratification, illuminated the mechanisms of self-control, and reframed my thinking around weight loss. You no doubt have heard of these strategies because psychologists use them all the time to treat many different conditions. You've just never seen them applied to food.

That amazing decrease of Oreo consumption from 16 to 3? The process is called 'habituation,' and it is standard treatment for prescription drug addiction.

My ability to dramatically cut back meal portions without feeling cheated? It's called 'systematic desensitization.' Psychologists use it to eliminate irrational fears and phobias.

My ability to resist temptation without that feeling of self-punishment or sacrifice? A well-known delayed gratification technique called, "If-Then Implementation Planning."

Academics, researchers and psychologists consider these techniques the gold standard for treating addictions and mastering self-control. But again, you've just never seen them applied to weight loss.

Basically, I took these proven approaches to self-control and modified them to reflect the unique physiological and psychological challenges to losing weight. In order to reference this constellation of psychological strategies and talk about them in easier ways to understand I named my approach, "The Scratch Plan." Named mostly because I wanted to scratch the word "diet" from my vocabulary.

The Scratch Plan allowed me to lose weight easily. To be clear, easy doesn't mean effortless. I put a lot of effort into it but there's a difference between effortful and painful. I didn't suffer. I didn't obsess. I wasn't anxious. It didn't hurt. I didn't feel cheated. Or felt that I sacrificed too much. I didn't have to shut my eyes and brace for impact every time I crossed paths with a bucket of fried chicken.

And neither will you.

There are a couple of things you should know about the Scratch Plan. It won't deprive you of favorite foods or force you to white-knuckle your way through 5-alarm cravings. But it does require patience. This is not a quick fix diet book. You're not going to lose 10 pounds in 10 minutes. It's going to take time. LOTS of time. WAY more time than you'd like. The Scratch Plan is not for people motivated by urgency; it's for people seeking permanence.

While I believe 'Scratch' can help everyone, even the most obese, I specifically aimed it at people who are "two weeks away from being fat" or only a few months into being overweight. Why? Because if you've been skinny or normal weight all your life, but suddenly start putting on pounds, you know it's possible to maintain weight without dieting (you've done it naturally all your life).

You're also much more receptive to the idea of moderation than chronically overweight folks because until recently, you've consistently exercised moderation (probably without knowing it). As a member of the 'about to get fat' or 'recently overweight' you're less likely to have the urgency that drives the chronically overweight into crash diets. This is important because you're not going to see results quickly.

You also are much less likely to *"eat your feelings."* Using food as a coping mechanism—eating to dull pain, frustration, anger, embarrassment, inadequacy, humiliation, or resentment presents a set of obstacles this book does not address.

Let's get back to those Oreos for a moment. Why did I stop at three? Why didn't I eliminate them from my diet altogether?

Because I didn't want to live in a world where I couldn't eat my favorite cookie. I didn't want to stop eating delicious foods (no matter how unhealthy); I wanted a way to control my eating so I could eat delicious foods AND lose/maintain my weight. I wanted moderation, not deprivation. And so should you. Eating tasty food—whether it's healthy fruit or an unhealthy basket of onion rings—is right up there with love and sex as Reasons To Live. Why would you cut yourself off from one of life's greatest pleasures? David Mamet once said, "We must have a pie. Stress cannot exist in the presence of a pie." I would amend that to say we must have naughty foods. Joy cannot exist in their absence.

Moderation doesn't mean eating tiny portions of whatever you want but leaving the table hungry. It means eating whatever you want but reducing the amount of food needed to

> Moderation doesn't mean eating tiny portions of whatever you want but leaving the table hungry. It means eating whatever you want but reducing the amount of food needed to make you feel full.

make you feel full. Today, I don't eat three Oreos at a sitting and force myself from the table, biting my fist and longing for the 16 I used to eat. I am as satisfied with three as I used to be with 16.

Moderation isn't about sacrificing satiety; it's about reducing the volume needed to reach satiety. But how do you get to moderation?

The secret to eating moderately is to make such gradual changes that your body doesn't notice it. Like a jet that imperceptibly turns left (as opposed to jerking the plane left and throwing the passengers against the walls), you make tiny reductions that the body can't react to (desensitization). You let your body acclimatize to the reduced level for a while (habituation). Once the reduced level becomes the body's 'new normal' you start another round of reductions. You keep doing this until you hit your target.

With that in mind, my plan will do three things for you:

Let You Eat Your Favorite Foods. There is nothing you can't have but you will have to put some rules around your choices. You're going to learn two innovative delayed gratification techniques that will make this possible. *Painlessly.*

Control Your Cravings. You will dramatically cut back the cravings of food or drink you consider unhealthy. Again, *painlessly.* If you're drinking 10 cans of Diet Coke a day I can get you to 1 or 2 without any withdrawals, constant cravings or will power fatigue.

Lose Weight Without Going On A Diet. You are not going to get a list of foods to eat or avoid. You are not going to get recipes or meal suggestions. I am not going to ask you to count calories, fat, carbs or sugar. I am not going to propose some wild new theory about weight gain. Those are all the marks of a diet and you are not going to go on a diet. You are going to permanently change the amount you eat, not what you eat. And you're going to do it with strategies identified by researchers and psychologists as the keys to self-control. Let me repeat that again:

*You are going to change how much you eat,
not what you eat.*

Keep The Dietary Restrictions You Must Or Want To Have. Are you a vegan or a vegetarian? Are you diabetic or allergic to gluten? Do you eat three meals a day or six? It doesn't matter because my plan does not require you to move toward or away from any particular foods or adhere to any kind of schedule. It's a self-control strategy not a dietary plan. You can apply these strategies to any food plan you want.

Use Your Definition Of "Healthy Foods" Not Mine. Again, my plan does not require you to eat or avoid any specific food though it does encourage choosing "healthy foods"—*however you define the term for yourself.* Vegans define 'healthy' differently than vegetarians who define it different-ly than meat-eaters who define it differently than gluten-free eaters. This is not a book that will tell you what foods to eat or avoid except in the most general terms. It is a book that will help you maintain or lose weight within the confines of whatever foods you think are healthy for you. My concepts for controlling cravings, for example, work just as well on Oreos as they do with any other food.

Improve Your Self Image. Not because you will lose weight—studies show that weight loss doesn't improve body image. Your body image will improve because you won't use the inevitable fall off a diet as a way to hate yourself and provide proof of personal failure. You will not 'punish' a misbehaving body for its lapses by taking it to the gym or the running track for an excruciating work out. You will not say things like, "I'm going to have to hit the gym extra hard after eating that dessert." Instead, you will say things like, "Wow, that was delicious. I can't wait to have that again sometime soon." You will see that the proper response to a fattening meal is to enjoy it, not to punish yourself for it.

A Sense Of Inner Peace And Calm About Food. Ever notice how people on a diet are constantly anxious about food? They are plagued by thoughts like, "I really want to eat that but it's not on my diet" and "If I eat that I will be a failure, a complete loser for not keeping to my diet." You will not experience that *because you won't be on a diet.* You will treat food as it is meant to be treated—as something to enjoy, without guilt or anxiety.

An Enhanced Sense Of Well-being. Food is so primal to our existence that your relationship to it reverberates in all aspects of your life. Food, or rather your relationship to it, can be a major life stressor. By eliminating the anxieties you have around it you will greatly improve your sense of well-being, which will positively affect other areas of your life—your relationships, work and over-all approach to living.

You have the ability to control your cravings and lose weight without giving up your favorite foods. It isn't about will power, it's about know how.

CHAPTER ONE

The Best Way To Lose Weight Is To Stop Dieting

Change How Much You Eat Without Feeling Deprived

If diets work why are there so many diet books? Why do so many people fail at it? Is it low will power? A lack of self-control? Are they choosing the wrong diets? With studies showing diets have a 95% failure rate you would probably agree with the scientific consensus that diets don't work.

Weight loss researchers have proved that dieting creates fat-promoting biological responses. The harder you try to reach your goal the harder your body fights back. Your goal (weight loss) is interpreted as a threat to your body's existence. It will literally slow down your metabolism to the point that you can get fatter on a lower intake of calories. It will also make you ravenously hungry—far hungrier than you were pre-diet.

This is the quandary that all dieters face: the very act of dieting creates an equal and opposing force to it. These two facts lay side by side and like Frida Kahlo's eyebrows, they cannot be separated. When you combine a significant increase in hunger with a significant decrease in metabolism you create the conditions for massive failure.

Our first order of business is to avoid these fat-promoting biological responses. We're going to do that with a number of psychological strategies but they will not work without a fundamental change in your consciousness. Namely, that you stop dieting. To understand why let's take a deeper look at the science behind your body's biological responses to restricted eating.

Dieting is about deprivation—you stop or severely restrict intake of certain foods. This deprivation triggers the body's fight or flight syndrome, which produces two unwelcome phenomenon: It slows the metabolism and dramatically increases cravings to the point that it overwhelms will power. Once that happens, psychologists refer to the consequences as the "Boomerang Effect"—you end up gaining back all the weight you lost, and in some cases, even more than before you started the diet.

Studies show that dieting triggers signals from the brain to increase fuel consumption (we get hungrier) and save energy (our metabolism slows down). The stricter the diet the more predictable the increases in hunger and slower metabolism. Here's a sample study (there are many) that illustrates the findings: Dr. Rudolph L. Leibel of Columbia University and his colleagues conducted studies on lean and obese people. They put them on a diet with the goal of losing 10 to 20 percent of their weight. They measured the subjects' biological responses and what do you think happened? Their hunger increased and metabolism plummeted. Leibel's studies, and others like it, confirm that dieting elicits obesity-promoting biological responses.

In other words, one of the fastest ways to gain more weight is to go on a diet.

What exactly sets off your body's fight or flight response? Unfulfilled cravings. From a primal standpoint your body does not make a distinction between denying yourself food that exists (by say, exercising extreme will power at a cruise ship buffet) and the inability to eat because food does not exist (you're in deserted island and there's not so much as a coconut to munch on).

Will power over available food or alarm over nonexistent food, it's all the same to your body—it isn't eating what it wants. So it sends out flares, screams "mayday!" and goes into lock-down mode. It'll make you hungrier to overcome the obstacle to available food (your will power) or so ravenous that you'll think of more clever ways to hunt or find food.

How Do You Lose Weight Without Going On A Diet?

The first step is to stop triggering the biological responses to dieting. But how do you lose weight without restricting or eliminating foods? By making weight loss the result of a bigger goal than dieting.

Let me illuminate this with a quick story about Apple founder

Steve Jobs. He once famously explained why Apple succeeded with iPod when Microsoft failed miserably with its version of a music player: "Our goal was to build an insanely great product," he said. "Their goal was to make money."

In other words, revenue wasn't Apple's goal just like I'm saying weight loss shouldn't be yours. And just as Apple's goal was creating a gorgeous product that *resulted* in revenue, I'm saying your goal should be something that *results* in weight loss.

But what should that goal be? Health. A sense of well-being. Enriching your life by eating a wide variety of delicious foods while building a strong, healthy body. This includes fat bombs that are hands-in-the-air fantastic and foods that should come with a Terror Warning level, like spinach.

If you take weight loss off the table and concentrate on changing your eating strategies to reflect abundance and health instead of limitation and restriction you will attain a greater sense of well-being.

Now, it's easy to see how abundance (eating whatever you want) avoids the body's fight-or-flight response, but how does that result in weight loss? Because we're going to use proven psychological strategies like systematic desensitization, habituation and delayed gratification techniques to eat anything we want *in moderation*.

We're going to keep the variety but reduce the volume.

We're going to change how much we eat *without feeling deprived*. We're going to reduce the amount we eat without any suffering. We're going to add healthy foods without feeling cheated.

Once you attain moderation, weight loss is not just possible but *inevitable*. I am the living example of that. I aimed higher than weight loss—improving the quality of my life (in part by introducing moderation to my eating habits)—and it resulted in a permanent decrease in my weight.

Did I want to lose weight? Of course. Just like Apple wanted to make money. But I realized dieting wouldn't work. What could I aim for that would *result* in weight loss? A better quality of life. Higher satisfaction around the things that food influences—energy, mood, attitude, contentment, optimism. I wanted to improve my physical and mental well-being.

This is how much more effective a well-being goal is than a weight loss goal: When I was 28 and bursting out of my size 34 waist onto a 36, I would have set my goal at losing only a few pounds. I simply wanted to stay at a size 34. But attaining my well-being goal resulted in a loss of 14 pounds and a reduction to a size 32 waist (and kept it that way for 25 years and counting). How is this possible?

I set up a more effective goal than dieting. When Steve Jobs aimed for beauty, design and functionality the market responded with money. When Microsoft aimed for money the market responded with financial calamity. It's the same with well-being—aim for it and the 'market' responds with weight loss. Aim for weight loss and the 'market' responds with an epic, waist-expanding fail.

Steve Jobs did not ask his team for an estimate of how much money the iPhone could make. That would be making money the goal, not the result. Instead, he asked them what kind of awesome things it should be able to do, how beautiful it could look, and how best it could help people's lives. That's a completely different goal…that resulted in a lot of money.

People almost always fail when they make weight loss the goal rather than the result of well-being. Take exercise, for example. Did you know that people who use exercise as a tool to lose weight are far more likely to stop than people who use exercise to enhance well-being (and lose weight as a result)? That's because dieters tend to look at exercise as a quick fix rather than a healthy activity and get disappointed when they don't see near instant results. They also don't realize that exercise makes you hungrier, making it harder to stick to a diet.

Studies also show that people who exercise to lose weight end up having a worse body image than people who exercise to be healthier. When you are constantly on a scale checking to see if exercise slimmed you down it reminds you how dissatisfied you are with your body.

Clearly, goals matter. A weight loss goal takes you in one direction; a well-being goal takes you to another. Here's a chart that compares the two:

	Goal: Lose Weight	Goal: A Sense Of Well-Being
Strategy	• Go on a diet. Restrict most foods and cut out whole categories (carbs, for instance).	• Change eating strategies to eat a wide variety of delicious foods (including fat and sugar bombs) while building a strong, healthy body. Use desensitization to dramatically reduce cravings for unhealthy foods and use pain-free delayed gratification techniques to moderate portions.
	• Set a weight loss goal: 5, 10 or 15+ pounds	• Set a psychological goal: Feel good, better or great.
Time Frame	• A week, a month, three months.	• No time frame. It's a way of life.
Monitoring Progress	• Weigh yourself daily or weekly.	• Never get on the scale for the first three months.
Questions You Ask Yourself	• Is this on my diet?	• Am I changing the way I eat without feeling deprived?
	• Should I eat this?	• Am I starting to eat less and

	Goal: Lose Weight	**Goal: A Sense Of Well-Being**
	• Am I losing weight fast enough? • How much time am I going to have to spend at the gym to work this off? • How long will I be able to keep this weight off?	less without any real suffering? • Am I adding more healthy foods without feeling cheated? • Am I seeing measurable progress in cutting back "Oreos" (or whatever your problem food is) with the desensitization method? • What's on TV?
State Of Mind	• Constantly anxious about making the right food choices. • 24/7 vigilance about "staying on the diet." • Deteriorating self-image (Every time you go off your diet you beat yourself up for having no will power, no discipline).	• Completely calm and at ease about food choices. • What's on TV? • Enhanced self-image. You're having a blast eating foods you LOVE while learning new strategies for choosing healthier foods. You see the slow-but-permanent results and it makes you feel good about yourself.
Weight Loss	• Lose weight rapidly	• Lose weight slowly

	Goal: Lose Weight	Goal: A Sense Of Well-Being
	• Regain the weight as soon as the diet ends (because you've *temporarily* changed the foods you eat).	• Keep the weight off forever (because you've *permanently* changed *the way* you eat).

Set The Right Expectation.

It's going to take time. Not a little time. A LOT. One of the great themes you'll see permeating this book is the idea of slow, gradual change. This amounts to heresy in a land that looks for instant results, but you can give in to urgency or reach for permanence.

It took me about six months to lose 14 pounds and almost two pant sizes. That's a half a pound a week! That's a long time compared to diets. But again, I want to remind you, I wasn't on a diet. And the best part, again, is that *my weight and pants size has remained constant for 25 years* without suffering any deprivation or exercising white-knuckled will power.

And here's the mind-blowing part: I don't cook. I go out to eat for at least half my meals. I tried to cook when I first started The Scratch Plan but I ended up using the smoke alarm as a timer. Even the dog didn't like my cooking. I'd give him a bite and he'd lick his butt to get the taste out of his mouth.

My point is that is that I would have lost even more weight if I lived in a household where somebody cooked, because you almost always eat healthier at home than at restaurants.

"God, Grant Me Patience. But Hurry!"

What if you're obsessed with losing weight quickly? This happens a lot to people who have important events coming up—a high school reunion, a keynote speech, a pending beach vacation. The urgency to lose weight quickly is real and profound, and unfortunately aided and abetted by the weight loss industry.

You have to come to terms with the fact that you won't lose weight quickly on The Scratch Plan. One way of managing the urgency (especially if you have an important event coming up) is to go ahead and pick a diet that will help you lose weight quickly. It will, of course be unsustainable and you will soon regain the weight. At that point, you will be far more receptive to the question I pose to you: Would you rather have a quick but temporary loss of ten pounds or a slow but permanent one?

When I first started down this road I realized early on that I had to let go of the desire for quick results. I realized I couldn't be 'involved' in a long-term strategy; I had to be committed. And if you don't know the difference between involvement and commitment let me spell it out for you. It's like an eggs and bacon breakfast: The chicken was involved. The pig was committed.

The Scratch Plan does not ask you to suffer but it does ask for your commitment. You will not succeed if you let your short-term desires get in the way of longer-term outcomes. Commit yourself to permanence and the urgency will recede.

Now That You're Not On A Diet, Stop Acting Like You Are.

Although you are going to make changes to the way you eat you have to "prove" to your body that you're not on a diet. It's only when your body is convinced that its survival is not at stake that it will stop its fat-promoting biological responses and allow you to make the changes that result in weight loss.

You must move your body from a Fight Or Flight response to a Relax & Unwind repose. The best way to do that is to cultivate an attitude of "plenty" not "lack" in your food choices. Your new mentality is simple and understood by the body: *"I am going to eat whatever I want. There is nothing I can't have."* Pizza? Done. Ice cream? Check. Steak? High Five. Nothing is off-limits. As you'll soon see, there will be limitations to portions and frequency but for now, it's critical to shift from a restrictive consciousness of food (diet) to an unlimited one (well-being). That means honoring your body's cravings—whether they are healthy or not.

Say Goodbye To Punishing Or Rewarding Yourself With Food.

Cottage cheese is to food what painting by numbers is to art: A weak imitation unworthy of your attention. Dieters eat it to "punish" themselves into weight loss. And after eating enough of the albino paste they "reward" themselves at the end of the week with a tub of Ben & Jerry's Phish Food (my personal fave!). This is typical of a dieter's mentality: Tough it out with punishing foods and then reward yourself with an oasis of taste. There is no place for that type of thinking in the Scratch plan. There are no "rewards" in a consciousness of plenty. They are just part of the landscape, or if you will, the picnic table. I never, EVER, say to myself, "I'm going to reward myself this weekend with naughty food." I eat naughty food on a regular basis.

> ## If You Do Not Punish Your Body
> ## You Do Not Need To Reward It.

If you do not grasp this concept—that you are not going on a diet; that you are going on a journey of well-being—you will be doomed to failure because you will set off your body's biological responses to dieting—more hunger and a slower metabolism. Besides, food is not there to punish or reward you. It is there to sustain you. To nourish you. To make you whole.

Forget Setting Weight Loss Goals Like "I Want To Lose 10 Pounds."

Do not set a weight loss goal. That's a diet mentality. Set a well-being goal. That's a quality of life mentality. Your goal is an enhanced sense of well-being. Your goal is to feel good, better or best, not to lose 5, 10 or 15 pounds. The minute you say something like, "I want to lose 10 pounds" you've adopted a diet goal. You will make food choices on the basis of whether it will help you lose weight not whether you like it, want it or think it will improve your sense of well-being. Bad move, because soon your body will learn it is, in fact, on a diet, and it will trigger the obesity promoting biological responses we're trying to avoid.

Now, I don't want to be stupid about this. You would not have bought this book if you didn't have a burning desire to lose weight. I'm not saying you shouldn't *want* to lose weight. I'm saying you shouldn't set it as a goal.

Hide Your Scale.

Do not weigh yourself. That's what a dieter does to check his or her progress. It's fine to check—*against the right goal.* Your goal isn't to lose weight—it's to enhance your well-being. So if you want to check your progress, don't step on a scale, ask yourself some crucial questions:

- Am I changing the way I eat without feeling deprived?

- Am I starting to eat less and less without any real suffering?

- Am I adding more healthy foods without feeling cheated?

- Am I seeing measurable progress in cutting back "Oreos" (or whatever your problem food is) with the desensitization method?

If the answer is "Yes" then your progress is good. If the answer is "No" then check back with these chapters and make sure you're following the instructions.

I recommend checking your weight about three months after implementing this plan. Then you can check whenever you want as often as you want. Steve Jobs checked his sales figures all the time—but only AFTER his higher-mission goal was achieved. At the end of three months you will have achieved enough progress against your well-being goal to measure the results.

From Vicious Cycle To Virtuous Circle.

Upgrading your goal from weight loss to well-being lifts you from the vicious cycle of dieting to the virtuous circle of health:

Vicious Cycle

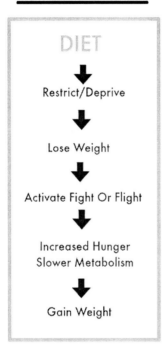

DIET
⬇
Restrict/Deprive
⬇
Lose Weight
⬇
Activate Fight Or Flight
⬇
Increased Hunger
Slower Metabolism
⬇
Gain Weight

Virtuous Cycle

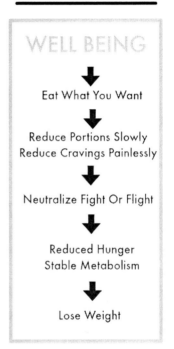

WELL BEING
⬇
Eat What You Want
⬇
Reduce Portions Slowly
Reduce Cravings Painlessly
⬇
Neutralize Fight Or Flight
⬇
Reduced Hunger
Stable Metabolism
⬇
Lose Weight

Good To The Last Thought.

A senior citizen was wondering if his wife had a hearing problem. So one night, he stood behind her while she was sitting in her lounge chair. He spoke softly to her. *"Honey, can you hear me?"*

There was no response. He moved a little closer and said again, *"Honey, can you hear me?"* Still, no response.

Finally he moved right behind her and said, *"Honey, can you hear me?"*

She replied, *"For the third time, YES!"*

I know I'm saying this for the third time, but I want to make sure that you can hear me loud and clear: YOU ARE NOT ON A DIET. You are on a journey toward well-being.

At this point, you're probably wondering how in God's pajamas you're going to lose weight if you can eat anything you want.

Let's find out.

Where Are We?

We shifted our goal from weight loss to well-being. We are not on a diet; we are on a journey to well-being, which results in weight loss.

We avoid triggering the body's fat-promoting biological responses to dieting. We don't restrict or ban foods, set weight loss goals, or weigh ourselves constantly.

CHAPTER TWO

Stop Binging With Systematic Desensitization

How I Went From Eating 16 Oreos To 3
Without Missing The 13 In Between

A consciousness of plenty applies to variety not volume. You have to honor your new consciousness of well-being by eating a wide variety of foods—basically anything that tastes good to you (whether it's healthy or not). But you're going to temper it by controlling the amount you eat along with the frequency with which you eat it.

It's been a long-held conclusion by research scientists that variety and moderation are the keys to weight loss success because they completely neutralize the fight or flight response. They also satisfy the human inclination toward the tasty. But moderation, also known as portion control, has its own demons. In fact, scientists have found that people have a harder time exercising moderation than deprivation.

In other words, most people would find it easier to give up ALL my Oreos than to go from eating 16 to eating three. Of course, within a couple of months they'd be right back to eating the 16 and possibly more.

Why is moderation harder than deprivation? This question stumped researchers until they observed an interesting phenomenon: Most people use deprivation techniques to reach moderation.

In other words, when people try for moderation they don't just "cut back" they *dramatically* cut back. So severely that their bodies lurch into a fight or flight response equivalent to full-on deprivation. Their metabolism slows and their cravings roar.

How Not To Achieve Portion Control

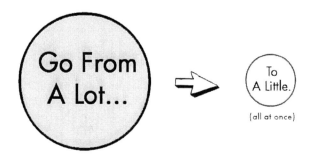

I bet when I told you that I went from eating 16 Oreos to three you thought I immediately cut 13 Oreos from my portions. In fact I did no such thing. I cut back so gradually that I never triggered my body's fight or flight response. Actually, I did it so gradually my body didn't even notice I was doing it.

The key to achieving portion control isn't to go from large to small. It isn't even to go from large to medium. It's to go from large to a hair smaller than large. And from there to a hair smaller than that. Rinse, lather, repeat. You keep making tiny reductions until you get to a serving size that makes sense—without ever throwing your body into fight or flight or triggering uncontrollable cravings.

Psychologists have labels for this process: 'Systematic desensitization' and 'habituation.' You make tiny reductions that the body can't react to (desensitization). You let your body acclimatize to the reduced level for a while (habituation). Once the reduced level becomes the body's 'new normal' you start another round of reductions. You keep doing this until you hit your target. And by the time you hit your target your body doesn't know what hit it.

Systematic desensitization and habituation are the principal methods psychologists and psychiatrists use to treat prescription drug addiction. If these processes get people off Vicodin imagine how well they'll work on getting you off potato chips.

The body resists sudden, dramatic changes but adapts easily to small, almost imperceptible ones. Think of your body's response to "cutting back drastically" as if it were a jet plane that makes a sudden 90-degree turn at 600 MPH—the people in the cabin scream, panic, cry, and pray as everything that isn't bolted down flies across the seats (including the passengers). Even after the plane straightens out, panic remains. Compare that to the plane turning one degree at a time. Yes, it takes a lot longer, but you'll get there in time and the passengers are calm, happy and look forward to the next trip.

Obviously, making almost imperceptible reductions in the portions you eat requires time—a LOT of time. But one thing it does not require is pain.

Remember my friend Mike, the editor of a health magazine that vetted weight loss studies? He's the one who bet that he could drastically reduce my intake of Oreos without any wild cravings or the feeling of unendurable sacrifice that usually accompanies deprivation. I'm happy to say he won the bet, so let me show you how he guided me through the desensitization and habituation.

From 16 to 3. How To Stop Overeating Your Favorite Food.

As you read the process I used to dramatically reduce my Oreo intake I invite you to think of your own "problem food" that you're eating too much of.

While I am a little leery of equating my craving for sugar with an addict's craving for drugs, there is no question that systematic food desensitization works through the same principle—"habituating" the body to smaller and smaller dosages of the craved substance without triggering 'withdrawal symptoms' (in our case, the body's fat-promoting biological responses).

Systematic desensitization for food requires a sensible withdrawal schedule. In other words, you are going to taper off the "drug" in such small incremental drops that your body can hardly perceive what you're doing.

How Much Of The Problem Food Are You Eating?

When Mike asked me how many Oreos I was eating at a sitting I told him I didn't know. I just kept eating until I didn't want anymore. I'd reach into the pack as I was watching a game and hoover them. All I knew was that the package looked like a linebacker hit it when I was done.

This was my first lesson in systematic desensitization: Know thy number. You can't reduce your intake if you don't know what you're taking in.

So here's what Mike made me do. He made me count the number of Oreos I was popping into my mouth. I was shocked when I realized that I typically ate 16 Oreos at a sitting. *Shocked.* Because I never really paid attention—especially when my team was at the ten-yard line with one down and two to go. I just assumed I ate, well, not a LOT but you know, a lot-ish. Well, there is no "-ish" in 16 Oreos. That's Type 1 diabetes arm-wrestling Type 2 for a shot of insulin.

Be that as it may, we had a number to measure progress from: 16 Oreos.

Warning: Do Not Awaken The Body's Fat-Producing Biological Responses.

When Mike guided me through the process, his first piece of advice was to make sure that my body didn't freak out at the reduction of Oreos he proposed. The best way to do that he said, was for me to reduce the number of Oreos so slightly that my body would have a hard time perceiving the difference.

We were sitting at my kitchen table with a package of Oreos when Mike asked me to turn around so I wouldn't see what he was doing. "Okay," he said as he shook the Oreos out of the box and arranged them on two plates. "On a count of three I want you to turn around and give me your reaction.

One.

Two.

Three."

This is what I saw:

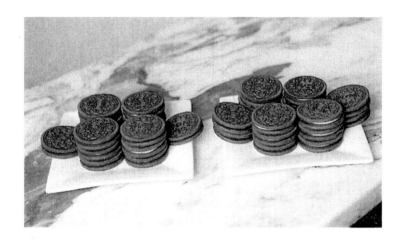

"Which plate has the most Oreos?" Mike asked.

I paused for a moment because at first both plates looked about equal. Then I saw the difference and pointed to the one on the right.

"Exactly," said Mike. "Now, take a look at this drawing and tell me, on a scale of 1 to 10, your reaction to eating the plate with 14 Oreos rather than the one with 16."

The drawing looked something like this:

Craving Intensity
Spectrum

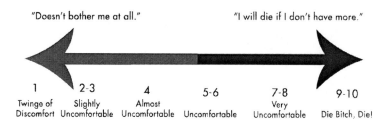

"Doesn't bother me at all."   "I will die if I don't have more."

1	2-3	4	5-6	7-8	9-10
Twinge of Discomfort	Slightly Uncomfortable	Almost Uncomfortable	Uncomfortable	Very Uncomfortable	Die Bitch, Die!

"It's really important that you don't intellectualize this exercise," Mike said. "Don't tell me what you think I want to hear or what you think it "should" be or what you want it to be. I'm not looking for your opinion but your *reaction*.

I looked at the chart and said, "Almost zero anxiety." I had such a hard time making a distinction between the two piles that I honestly didn't believe there was much difference. Now, if I had seen two piles like *this* it would have been a completely different story:

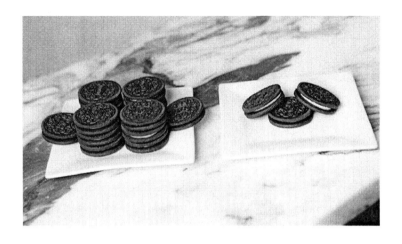

In that case, I would have said my anxiety was a 10 out of 10. But instead, the piles Mike set out for me looked so similar I almost couldn't tell the difference.

Mike handed me the plate with the 14 Oreos and said, "Knock yourself out." So I did. I ate all 14 cookies. After I was done he asked me a simple question: "On a scale of 1 to 10, how intense is your craving to eat the two additional Oreos you would have normally eaten?" I said, "Around a 2."

Now, I don't want to mislead you. I would have *preferred* to have the other two Oreos (to make it to the 16 I would have normally eaten) but I didn't feel the *need* for them. It wasn't painful to deny myself the other two Oreos, just slightly uncomfortable. This was a key concept that Mike helped me grasp. Portion reduction does not require pain. In fact, pain (defined as the intensity of your craving) is the enemy. Pain is the signal that you've cut your portions too much too soon.

Mike's next instructions took me by surprise. I thought for sure he was going to tell me that I should cut my next Oreo feeding down to 12 cookies. Instead, he made me promise that I would not cut my intake from 14 cookies. "I want you to stay at 14 cookies for the next two or three times you decide to chow down on them." For the record I did not eat 16 Oreos a day. I ate that much about twice a week. You think I was that big of a pig? Geez.

Impatient, I asked Mike why I couldn't simply eat 12 Oreos the next time I pigged out. "I had very little problem going from 16 to 14," I said. "Why would I have a problem going from 14 to 12?" Mike likened it to deep-sea divers descending to the ocean floor. "Once you descend to a new depth you must get your body used to the pressure or you'll start getting the bends. It's the same with reducing cravings," he said. "You're going to stay at 14 cookies to stabilize your body so that it sees 14 as the new normal."

In other words, he proposed a sensible withdrawal schedule.

I did as Mike said and I ate 14 Oreos the next few times that I had a craving for them. I called Mike and said, "Okay, I'm pretty sure 14 is now my new normal. What's next?"

Mike came over with a bag of Oreos and once again asked me to turn my back. I could hear him set up two plates of Oreos and when I turned around I saw this:

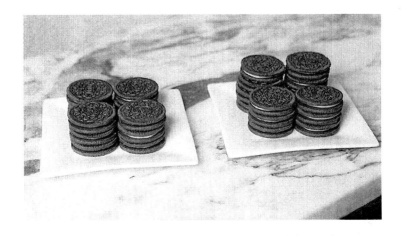

Again, there was a momentary pause, as the pile count seemed similar at first glance.

Once I identified the 12-Oreo pile Mike asked me to rate, on a scale of 1 to 10, my anxiety of choosing the pile with the fewer Oreos. I told him it was about a 1 (a twinge of discomfort). Mike said as long as I was within the 1 to 3 range I should allow myself to eat the pile with the least amount of cookies. His rationale was simple: "Slightly uncomfortable is manageable." I ate all 12 cookies. When I was done Mike asked me the familiar question—how badly did I want to eat the remaining two Oreos? My answer was "Low. Very low."

"Cool," he said. "Just remember that once you get up to "medium or high" it means you underestimated your craving and should go ahead and eat the remaining cookies. This isn't about depriving yourself to the point of pain. It's about depriving yourself to the point of no pain. Or rather, so little pain you don't really mind.

Getting The Food "Bends."

Mike recommended that I stick to 12 Oreos for the next three or four "feedings" and that's what I did. I repeated Mike's systematic desensitization process without any problems until I "descended" to eight cookies at a sitting. For whatever reason, my anxieties shot up to a seven or eight when I doled out the cookies. "Go up to 10 cookies," Mike said, "and stay there for a few feedings."

Of course I felt like a complete failure because suddenly my downward trajectory was derailed. "Nonsense," said Mike. "Divers get the bends at different depths. Just because somebody's tolerance level is higher or lower doesn't make them a better or worse diver. They just have to acclimate themselves better. You got the food "bends" at a depth you hadn't expected. All that means is that you need to go to a shallower depth, stay there to acclimatize yourself, and then drift downward."

So that's what I did—I went up to 10 cookies and stayed there for the next few feedings. In a couple of weeks I went down to eight cookies with almost zero level discomfort. In fact I was so elated I called Mike up and told him I was going to go down to four Oreos at my next feeding. "Bad move," he said. Do NOT do that. Do you know what they call deep-sea divers who descend too quickly?" he asked. "DEAD IN THE WATER."

Mike was absolutely insistent that I descend slowly even if I felt okay with speeding it up. I stuck with eating eight Oreos at a time for the next few feedings. From there I went to six.

Now, a funny thing happened when I got to six Oreos. My anxieties flared up and I had to go up to 8 cookies per feeding. Mike had an idea: Instead of dropping two cookies at a time, drop one. It worked. I went from 8 to 7 without a problem. And then from 7 to 6.

Getting stuck on 8 cookies illuminated a central premise about desensitization/habituation: When in pain, extend the habituation and slow the descent. Time is your friend; impatience is the enemy.

From there, it was only a matter of a few more weeks before I got down to three Oreos.

Three Oreos!

I couldn't believe it. I went from pigging out on 16 Oreos at a time to eating three without suffering more than a twinge of discomfort. Mike had taught me the secret to dramatically cutting back on problem foods: A slow, gradual descent from one "depth" to the next without triggering "the bends."

So was I able to keep myself to three Oreos? Funny you should ask. Because the truth is that after a while I stopped eating Oreos altogether. Why? Part of it is due to a well-documented phenomenon: Sugar creates more craving for sugar. Conversely, the less you have it the less you want it.

My cravings for Oreos simply weakened to the point that it was as easy not to have them as it was to reach for them. Don't get me wrong, I still occasionally indulge, but they're not the "must" they once were. They have almost no power over me. Now, "the less you have it the less you want it" phenomenon is only part of the reason why I stopped eating Oreos. The real reason I stopped is that I, well, let's save that for the next chapter, where the context will make more sense.

Enough About Me. Let's Talk About You.

Let's go over the process of systematic desensitization/habituation as applied to your particular problem food. It's easy to do it with foods that come in standard sizes (cookies, candy, beverages, etc.) because they're packaged in units that are easily measured. But treats like potato chips, cakes, pies, and ice cream are a little bit harder because you're pretty much eyeballing the portions you serve yourself. For example, if your problem food is potato chips (and really, whose isn't?) then conducting a desensitization/habituation 'descent' will be more difficult. What are you going to do—count out potato chips? I think not.

Still, you have to know how much you're eating in order to put a system around decreasing its intake. You cannot avoid triggering your body's fight or flight response with a desensitization program unless you know what your body considers a "normal" amount of the food.

Let's say you know you're eating way too many potato chips but you don't actually know how much because you eat them straight from a family-sized bag (oh, you naughty thing!). Believe me, I know how that works. You innocently start eating a few chips, go through the whole bag, and the next thing you know you've got the clerk at the QuikTrip in a headlock because they ran out.

If desensitization and habituation get people off Vicodin, imagine how well they'll work on getting you off potato chips.

The first rule of holes applies here—if you're in one, stop digging. DO NOT EAT OUT OF THE BAG. This is actually a simpler habit to break than you think. It's not painful, just mindful. You are going to eat what your body craves; just not in the mindless way you're used to. There is a big difference between inconvenience and deprivation. So while you may think it's a bummer to stop eating out of the bag, take comfort in the fact that you're still getting the goods. So, let's find out how many potato chips you're eating. I want you to go out and buy a food scale, a family-sized bag of potato chips and plastic sandwich bags.

I'll wait.

Back already? Great. I hope you paid cash or I may have to wean you off credit cards like Mike weaned me off Oreos.

Anyway, the next time you have a craving for chips I want you to put the unopened bag, the food scale and the sandwich bags in front of you. Put the bag of chips on the scale and jot down how much it weighs (I know it tells you on the bag, but I want to confirm it).

Next, start eating out of the bag until you are satisfied. Don't be all judgmental about how much you're eating. *EAT.* Mangia, mangia. Enjoy it. Stop only when your body truly has had enough. Not when you think you should (as in "I should stop—I'm a pig"), but when you are completely sated (as in "I no longer crave potato chips"). Think of it as taking your "Potato chip temperature." You're just determining how much you're eating.

Once you are completely sated, put the bag on the food scale and weigh it. Let's say the bag weighed 13.5 oz. when you started and now it weighs 9.5 oz. Congratulations! You just found out how many potato chips you eat at a sitting— 4 oz.—or four times the ordinary 1 oz. serving.

Admittedly, finding out how many potato chips you eat at a sitting can be misleading. After all, your cravings most likely fluctuate—sometimes they're overwhelming and you eat a lot and sometimes they're not so you don't.

That's why you need to do this measurement several times to establish your baseline. Remember, when Mike asked me how many Oreos I ate at a sitting I flat-out didn't know. He asked me to count my next three feedings and get an average. That's how I came upon the number of 16. The truth is I sometimes ate 14 and sometimes 18.

Go ahead and "take your potato chip temperature" a couple of more times. For the sake of simplicity, let's say you average 4 oz. of potato chips per feeding. Now get ready to…

Eat A Whole Lot Less Potato Chips Without Any Pain or Suffering.

Here are the steps to desensitizing yourself to eating fewer potato chips and habituating to the new reduced level without suffering any pain:

1) **Pour 4 oz. Into Sandwich Bag #1.** Place it on the counter.

2) **Pour 4 oz. Into Sandwich Bag #2.** Place it so that the bags are side-by-side.

3) **Reduce The Number Of Chips In Bag #2.** Take

out about 10-15% worth of potato chips. Then close your eyes and move the bags around so you don't know which bag is bigger.

4) **Compare.** Which bag has the smallest amount of potato chips?

5) **Rate Your Anxiety.** How much pain are you in at the thought of eating the smaller bag?

6) **Eat If The Anxiety Is Low, Add If It's High.** Low? Mangia! High? Add a few more chips until you only feel mild discomfort.

7) **Habituate.** Stay at the reduced level of chips for the next few feedings until it becomes the new normal.

8) **Desensitize.** Start a new round of reductions using the same steps outlined above.

9) **Keep Going Until You Hit Your Target.** Your target should never be zero—that would be deprivation. Your target should be moderation—around a 1 oz. serving.

Just to be clear, let's retrace our steps:

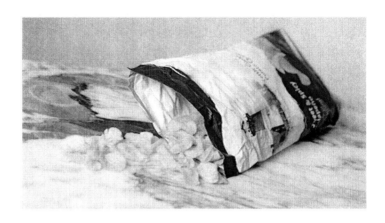

Buy It.

Make sure it's a family-size bag. They're usually 10.5 to 13.5 ounces or more. I want you eating out of a big bag, not a single portion bag.

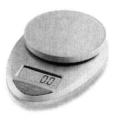

Weigh It.

Use a food scale. Make sure it's sensitive enough to measure ounces.

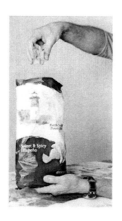

Eat It.

Pig out. Do not feel guilty. Eat until completely satisfied. You're taking your "Potato Chip temperature."

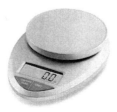

Weigh It Again.

Weigh the same bag you just ate out of. The difference between the before and after weight will determine the size of your "feeding." Let's say the bag weighed 13.5 oz. before you pigged out and 9.5 oz. afterwards. That means you typically eat 4 oz. of potato chips when you pig out on them.

Pour

Pour 4 oz. of potato chips into two plastic storage bags. That is, 4 oz. into the first bag, then 4 oz. into another. You should have two bags with the same amount of potato chips in them.

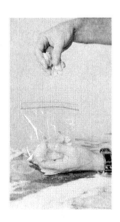

Subtract

Take 12-15% out of one of the bags. Twelve percent of 4 oz. would be .48 oz. Make sure you weigh it to get an exact measurement.

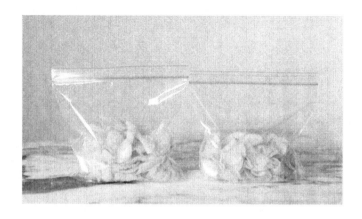

Compare

Compare the two bags. You should have a momentary pause of indecision before correctly identifying the bag with fewer potato chips. You're aiming for a barely perceptible reduction to avoid the body's fight or flight response.

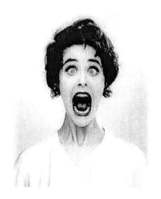

Rate Your Anxiety

How anxious are you about eating the smaller bag of potato chips versus the larger one? Use a 1-10 scale, ten being the highest level of anxiety. If you're above "3" put more chips in the smaller bag. Pain is a signal that you've reduced too much.

And there you have it—your first potato chip reduction! Eat. Enjoy. And follow this same process for the next round of reductions, always remembering that you want barely perceptible reductions throughout your "descent." When do you stop? When you've reached moderation, not deprivation. Typically, that means a reasonable portion—about 1 oz.

Some Last Notes.

You can use this desensitization process for cakes and pies, too. If eating too much cake is a problem for you, simply weigh how much you eat at a single sitting and use that to benchmark your "descent."

Do not fall into the trap of trying to "eyeball" your portions. Systematic desensitization requires precision. It only works when you can mathematically measure your progress. Estimates will sabotage your success because you will guess wrong. People are generally terrible at estimating portion size.

It's also important to make visual, side-by-side comparisons of your portions all the way through the desensitization process. When it comes to food, the brain reacts more powerfully to sights than thoughts. You will avoid the fight or flight response if your body can see the proposed reduction and react calmly to it.

If your body reacts negatively upon seeing the reduction in portion size do NOT try to rationalize or persuade yourself to go through with the desensitization. Simply increase the portion size. I cannot stress this enough: You must be able to look at the size of your new portion and remain calm. And by "remain calm" I don't mean talking yourself into calmness. I don't mean doing things to calm yourself, like progressive muscle relaxations or deep breathing. I mean the kind of calm that comes as a natural reaction to unthreatening stimuli.

Remember when my body freaked out at the eight Oreo level? I went up to 10 cookies. It is absolutely normal to have a jagged descent. Just like the only way to cure the beginnings of the bends is to rise to a shallower depth, the only proper way to calm your body's anxiety is to increase the portion level.

No one is timing you so don't feel pressured that you must accomplish this goal by a certain date. In fact, assigning a date for completion will completely work against you. First, that is a dieter's mentality. Second, you will pressure yourself to accept unworkable anxiety levels. Third, if you set up a date for completion and you don't meet it you will beat yourself up for it. Again that's a dieter's mentality not a consciousness of enhanced well-being.

If you're like me, your obsession with quick results will be replaced by a fascination with your body's reaction to nearly imperceptible food reductions. When I descended to a 10–cookie depth level I remember thinking, "Oh my God, this is really working! I am reducing my cookie intake without any pain!" It was at that point in my education that I had a profound realization: Eating strategies are more important than food plans.

How I Went From Drinking 36 Ounces of Coffee To 12 Without Missing The 24 In Between.

Systematic desensitization doesn't just work for fatty or sugary foods. It also works on anything you think is unhealthy. Take coffee, for example. A couple of cups a day is actually healthy for you. But 36 ounces? Not so much. I was jittery and suffered from stomach upset every morning. Before knowing about systematic desensitization I would just try to cut my coffee intake by half or more. That ended up giving me the famous caffeine withdrawal headaches. But I got smart and used the desensitization process. Here's what happened:

Date	Action	Notes
Day 1	I pegged my consumption at 36 ounces	I actually did not know how much I was drinking because I simply made a big pot and drank whatever I wanted. Using a process similar to the one explained above it became clear that I was regularly drinking 36 ounces at a sitting.
Day 2	Poured coffee into two pitchers. Pitcher A: 36 oz. Pitcher B: 34 oz.	I could hardly tell the difference between the two pitchers. I marked my anxiety about a "1" and proceeded to drink the 34 ounces.
Day 3, 4, 5	I made and drank 34 ounces of coffee each morning.	I stayed at this level for three days to acclimate my body to the new normal of 34 oz.
Day 6	Poured coffee into two pitchers. Pitcher A: 34 oz. Pitcher B: 32 oz.	I could hardly tell the difference between the two pitchers. I marked my anxiety about a "1 or 2" and drank the 32 ounces.
Day 7, 8, 9	I made and drank 32 ounces of coffee each morning.	I let my body acclimatize to the new normal of 32 oz.

Day 10	Poured coffee into two pitchers. Pitcher A: 32 oz. Pitcher B: 30 oz.	For some reason, my body freaked out—a "7" on the anxiety scale. So I went back to 32 oz. I did not beat myself up for "failing." I realized that a jagged descent is normal.
Day 11, 12, 13, 14	I stayed at 32 oz.	
Day 15	Poured coffee into two pitchers. Pitcher A: 32 oz. Pitcher B: 30 oz.	This time my body did not react negatively so I went with 30 oz.
Day 16, 17, 18	Stayed at 30 oz.	…Until my body got used to routinely drinking 30 oz.
Day 19	Poured coffee into two pitchers. Pitcher A: 30 oz. Pitcher B: 28 oz.	My anxiety level was fine so I drank the 28 oz.
Day 20, 21	Stayed at 28 oz.	

Day 22	I was so used to the process I no longer needed the visual aid of pouring coffee into two pitchers so I could see the difference. I simply made 26 oz. of coffee that morning.	After a while you'll notice that you don't need visual aids to determine your anxiety levels. You can simply pose a question to yourself. In my case, I asked, "How anxious am I about drinking 26 ounces of coffee?" The answer was "not very" so I proceeded.
Day 23, 24, 25	I stayed at 26 oz.	
Day 26	I poured 24 oz. and stayed at that level for the next 3 days.	
…Through Day 45	I continued until I reached the 12 oz. level.	At that point I stopped the desensitization process. I didn't want to stop drinking coffee altogether. I just wanted to drink enough to avoid the jitters and the stomach upset. Mission accomplished!

Benefits To Systematic Desensitization.

The biggest benefit to desensitization is an enhanced sense of well-being. For example, reducing my Oreo intake from

16 to 3 dramatically cut back the amount of sugar I was putting in my body. I don't mind telling you that after I ate 16 Oreos at a sitting I experienced wild mood swings caused by the avalanche of sugar and my body's release of insulin to counteract it. After I reduced my consumption to three Oreos at a sitting I pretty much eliminated the mood swings, retaining a strong sense of calm and composure. I could concentrate much better and eliminated a lot of stress from my body.

Another great benefit to systematic desensitization is that you never long for what you've eliminated. For example, I don't miss the 13 Oreos I cut out from my feedings. I don't miss the 24 ounces of coffee that I cut out from my morning ritual. I don't walk around obsessing about the missing cookies or the absent caffeine. What explains this absence of loss? Again, psychologists call it "habituation." Desensitization done right habituates your body to the new normal. In other words, I have the same sense of satisfaction eating three Oreos that I once had eating sixteen.

This was a huge revelation for me—the experience of being just as satisfied with three Oreos as I was with 16—because it cemented my conviction that I was on the right path. See, like most people, I thought, "eating moderately" was code for "you'll never feel full again." I thought portion control meant pain management. I thought volume reduction meant perpetual dissatisfaction. I was wrong. Instead of experiencing loss and longing I experienced satiety and satisfaction.

Habituation has its own benefits. Once I habituated to three Oreos I felt like my stomach literally shrank. Today, I am physically unable to eat 16 Oreos at a time. The idea actually makes me a little nauseous. The same goes for coffee. If I drank 36 ounces today I'd be climbing the walls (when I wasn't sitting on the toilet). "Stomach shrinking" paid a lot of dividends as I moved to moderate my meal portions.

With systematic desensitization and habituation I moved closer to my goal of an enhanced sense of well-being and what was the result? *Weight loss.* When I cut my Oreo and coffee intake I also cut the carbs, calories and fat that come from so many cookies and coffee cream (you should have seen how much half and half I used on 36 ounces of java!).

How much weight did I lose? I couldn't begin to tell you. I didn't allow myself to get on a scale for three months. All I knew was that my pants were no longer tight and I hadn't even begun to employ the eating strategies you're about to read.

Where Are We?

We shifted our goal from weight loss to well-being. We are not on a diet; we are on a journey to well-being, which results in weight loss.

We avoid triggering the body's fat-promoting biological responses to dieting. We don't restrict or ban foods, set weight loss goals, or weigh ourselves constantly.

We use pain-free systematic desensitization techniques to reduce or eliminate binging. The reduction of sugar and fat enhances our sense of well-being, which results in weight loss.

CHAPTER THREE

Eat Healthier Without Forcing Yourself To Eat What You Don't Like

A Neat Trick To Eating Healthier Without Sacrificing Taste: "The Nutrilicious"

When I tell people I've kept off 14 pounds and nearly two waist sizes for 25 years by eating anything I want they look at me like they're watching a foreign film without subtitles. When they snap out of it, they typically ask the wrong question. Like, "How can you lose weight eating high calorie foods?" That's a dieter's mentality. The real question is how on earth are you going to get an enhanced sense of well-being if your diet consists of pizza and ice cream?"

The answer is to make eating healthy foods a priority. I love a burger, fries and a load of creamy coleslaw but if my goal is well-being then I know I can't have that five times a week. Later, I'm going to show you some clever strategies for restricting the frequency of "bad" meals without feeling cheated out of something you really want. For now let's concentrate on what I mean by eating healthy.

I am not going to tell you what foods you should eat or avoid because that's not what this book is about. You should have a pretty good idea of what this is *for you*. I am not, as a carnivore, going to tell a vegetarian what she should eat. I am not, as a cream-in-my-coffee-or-die kind of guy, going to tell a vegan that dairy is okay.

In fact, I think you should know something about me: I'm a nutritional illiterate. I don't know the difference between conventional and organic. I have no idea why I should pick whole grains over white bread except that I should. I haven't the foggiest about what's too much salt or sugar.

I'm also committed to my ignorance. *I don't want to know* how much protein is in one food versus how many carbs are in another or how much trans-fat is in something else. It bores me. I've got things to do, people to see and places to go. I've got bigger fish to fry and I don't care if it was farmed or line-caught.

You should feel relieved, not alarmed, by my unwillingness to tell you what to eat. You don't have to worry about following some esoteric food plan that may or not make sense to you. You don't have to worry about whether I got my science right or whether you agree with my nutritional recommendations or conclusions.

If I were to prescribe foods you would be on MY path to well-being rather than yours. Own your well-being. Don't outsource it—to me or anyone else. You have a unique constellation of likes (chocolate-covered apples? Really?), dislikes (no on KFC Extra Crispy? Off with your head!) and limitations (restricting salt for high blood pressure or sugar for diabetes). You are the best judge of what is healthy for you.

And if you're not, then become it. Do the research, ask the experts, weigh the evidence. There is a lot of contradictory data to most theories about what constitutes nutrition-rich foods. Aren't you glad I'm not adding to the confusion?

The Nutritional Goals I Set For Myself.

Still, it might be helpful for you to see how I approach eating healthy. I keep it simple. Stupidly simple. I consider a food to be healthy if it doesn't:

1. Come in a box.
2. Need to be defrosted.
3. Require a can opener.

In other words, fruits, vegetables, whole grains, and unprocessed meats and poultry are good; everything else is a varying degree of bad (and usually delicious). Almost everything science knows about healthy foods is based on those three factors. You don't need a detailed map to eat healthy; you need a basic compass. My three-criteria definition of healthy is due north. Just keep moving toward it.

What exactly does that mean? Add more fruits, vegetables, whole grains and unprocessed meats and poultry to your plate!

Correction.

Add more fruits, vegetables, whole grains and unprocessed meats and poultry *that you like*. We are not on a diet and we will not be forced to eat foods we don't like just because they're healthy. Don't like spinach? Screw it; don't eat it.

The Party Is In Your Mouth. Don't Ruin It With A Boring Guest List.

Succeeding with an I'm-not-on-a-diet-but-I-gotta-go-for-healthy mentality requires you to truly enjoy what you put in your mouth. Yes you have to party with a health purpose but the operative word here is "party," and you can't have a good one with a boring guest list.

Remember, half the fun of throwing a party is talking about whom you're *not* inviting. Don't invite foods with the personality of a Kansas zip code and think they'll mix well with foods realtors might describe as ocean-front property. Only invite the interesting with a wide variety of tastes, textures and smells. It is a mistake of monumental proportions to think that "balance" means eating foods you don't like because they're healthy and eating foods you love despite their unhealthiness. You can't just put a helping of raw cauliflower (ugh!) next to a portion of French fries (yay!) and call it a party. Like the dweebs and the jocks, they won't mix and nobody will have a good time. Especially the host.

My Secret To Eating Well: The "Nutrilicious."

I rarely eat anything on a regular basis just because it's healthy for me. It's like being on a diet—unsustainable. The only way I've been able to make eating healthy sustainable is to go for what I call the "Nutrilicious."

To me, foods can be categorized in two ways with varying gradations: Healthy-but-boring and unhealthy-but-exciting. The key to sustaining healthy choices is in the overlap between the two. Not a balance between the two; the overlap. Here, take a look:

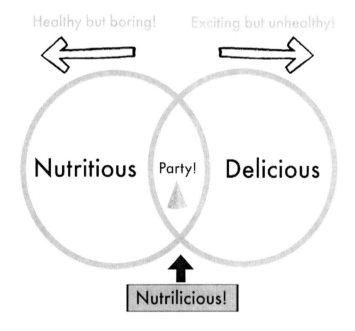

Nutrilicious foods are a fusion between healthy-but-boring and unhealthy-but-exciting. Let me give you an example: Raw broccoli. You just can't get healthier than that little bugger. But boring? You fall asleep halfway through its name. A compromise would be to order broccoli instead of French fries with your hamburger. Yuck. I would rather remove my eyes with a spoon.

Remember,, we're not reaching for compromise: We're reaching for fusion. Let's stay with the lowly raw broccoli for a moment. I'm fairly neutral about the hardy green stuff but I eat it all the time because I've made it delicious *for me*. One day, I dipped some raw broccoli into my favorite fatty, sugary salad dressing (Kraft Catalina!) and off to the races I went. Loved it. And then I got the big idea of adding a few peanuts. Even better. And then I got the idea of adding cheese. Pow! To the moon!

Raw broccoli with peanuts, cheese, and fatty, sugary salad dressing. To me, that's a party! It's a fusion between healthy and unhealthy that spells out "Nutrilicious." Some may question how that combination could be considered the healthiest eating. After all, the fat content is through the roof. The packaged dressing is full of sugars and God knows what kind of chemicals. How is that the healthiest eating? It's not. So why do I consider it healthy? Let me tell you a quick story.

I once surveyed about a dozen fitness experts for a maga-zine article and asked them a simple question: "What is the single best exercise for your body?" The answers ran the gamut from squats to pushups, but one expert's reply captivated me: *"The best exercise is the one you'll do."*

Apply this to food. What good are the healthiest foods if you won't eat them? I mean, what if you just don't like spinach? It may be one of the most nutritionally-dense foods but it's pointless to put it on your menu if you can't stomach it. I do not eat healthy foods I do not like and you shouldn't either.

This is one of my fundamental concepts: The best healthy foods are the ones you'll eat.

Could I make my broccoli concoction healthier? Of course. I could replace the peanuts with the more nutritionally-dense Brazil nuts. I could replace the Kraft Catalina (gasp!) with extra virgin oil and organic vinegar. But then I wouldn't eat it. And what's the point of preparing the healthiest food if I won't eat it?

Use "Food Viagra" On Lifeless Meals.

Getting to Nutrilicious requires you to identify a nutritious food (broccoli) and add ingredients to make it delicious (Catalina dressing, peanuts, cheese). Think of those ingredients as "Food Viagra" and ask yourself: What can I sprinkle on this nutrition-packed food that would make me stand at attention?"

Getting to Nutrilicious is a custom job. Some people might call my broccoli salad a hit; others would give it a miss. The definition of Nutrilicious is a nutritionally dense vegetable or fruit sprinkled with "food Viagra" to make it appealing *to you*. It's a terrific way of making sure you consistently eat healthy foods in a sustainable way. In an enjoyable way. In a way that makes you look forward to eating healthier.

You will be amazed at how many fruits and vegetables you will eat if you find a way to make them delicious. Don't buy into the purist idea that eating healthy doesn't count unless every ingredient is pitch perfect. I promise you I eat more broccoli than anyone on a diet and I'm not on one.

Finding The Nutrilicious Or Making Your Own.

Sometimes you get lucky and find a food that is completely healthy and completely delicious. Bananas, for instance. I love them and I don't have to dress them up in any way to make them taste better.

The best healthy foods are the ones you'll eat.

Then there are foods that reach the 90% mark in the Nutrilicious department. Take almonds. I can't stand them raw. But roasted and salted? OMG. All day long.

Now, roasting them takes some of the nutrition away and

adding salt is not good for an American diet that is already drowning in it. But which would you rather have—somebody eating a nutritional power food like roasted, salted almonds on a regular basis or somebody who rarely eats raw almonds because they taste like wet cardboard?

Free your mind. Health will follow.

Replacing "Bad" Foods With The Nutrilicious.

One of the great things about having a Nutrilicious mentality is that it frees you from purist thinking. This, in turn, helps you replace "bad" foods easily. And by bad, I mean foods that are so health-poor they don't have two nutrients to rub together. For instance I often replace hyper-salted no-good-for-you croutons with roasted almonds. Not because they are healthier but because they taste better. Notice I said I "often" replace croutons. "Often", not "always." I love croutons. No way I'm giving them up. But when my craving for them is low (and I still want something crunchy) it's easy to replace them with almonds or peanuts —something much healthier.

The First Rule Of Eating Nutriliciously:
Tasty First, Healthy Later.

You have to serve two masters in your quest for a better sense of well-being: Your taste buds and your health. You often have to engage in shuttle diplomacy as they battle each other in the quest for supremacy. You must end this war once and for all by changing your role from peacemaker to kingmaker. You must anoint your taste buds as ruler of the land. I know that sounds like blasphemy but hear me out: You will never eat a lot of healthy foods if your taste buds are an unwilling partner. Your body will find a way to subvert you.

Now, does that mean your taste buds are in complete control? No. Just because you're in charge doesn't mean you don't take differing views into account. Let me tell you a quick story about a company I worked for that had an ingenious way of helping leaders make sound decisions. They had what they called a "must-consult" model: You're in charge but you must consult with key constituencies before you make a decision. You talk to everybody affected by the situation, synthesize their varying opinions, needs and desires, and come up with an *informed* decision. It guaranteed that you took other people's views into account before making a decision.

This is my guiding principle for finding and/or creating the Nutrilicious: Taste is large and in charge but it must consult with Health before making a decision.

Making Healthy Decisions Based On Taste.

I don't buy organic because I think it's healthier than conventional; I buy it because I can taste the difference. If I can't I won't shell out the bucks for it. This is a fundamental aspect of your success with The Scratch Plan: Do not eat healthy foods just because they're healthy or because you feel like you should or because you think you'll lose weight with them.

Eat them because they're delicious.

I love fried chicken. Extra crispy. I also love salads. With lots of dressing (Catalina anyone?). One is clearly healthier than the other. Yet, I look forward to both with almost equal intensity. Why? Because I figured out how to make my salads so tasty that they actually compete with my craving for fried chicken.

Beware The Health Nazis.

They're everywhere and their job is to make you feel guilty about your choices. It's one thing for somebody to point out the difference between healthy and unhealthy foods. Those are actually helpful people and you should listen to them. For example, it's useful to hear there is basically zero nutritional value to white bread and that you should choose a whole grain option instead. Or that iceberg lettuce is an empty nutritional vessel and that you're better off eating darker, nutrient-rich leafy greens.

But that's not what health Nazis do. Instead of encouraging you to switch from unhealthy to healthier foods, they berate you for choosing healthy over healthiest. Let me give you a perfect example. I love peanut butter. And there are many in scientific circles that believe peanut butter is the perfect food because it so wonderfully balances protein, carbs and fat. But I have a friend who crinkles her nose every time I pull out a jar of Jif peanut butter.

"Really?" she sniffs. "*Jif?*"

"Yeah," I say, "What's wrong with it?"

"Ugh. Do you know how many preservatives are in conventional peanut butter?" she asks. "They also have hydrogenated oils, sugar, salt, corn syrup and stabilizers."

She guilted me into buying an all-natural peanut butter. You know, the disgusting ones where the oil separates from the peanut butter. The kind that looks like the manufacturer tried to fart when it had diarrhea.

Have you ever tried to mix oil that separates itself from peanut butter? If spilling it all over the jar and the counter isn't bad enough (be a dear and hand me that towel) I beg you not to look at or taste the mixture, for your next visit to the toilet is going to look remarkably similar to what's in the jar.

My friend insisted that the slight taste difference and inconvenience of getting oil all over the counter was worth avoiding the supposed cancer-causing, hormone-shifting properties of conventional peanut butter.

Right.

This is what I mean by a health Nazi. It's the purist who bathes in the ecstasy of sanctimony. Somebody who sees healthy food in stark, black and white terms. You are either eating something healthy or you're going to burn in a cancerous hell for all eternity.

Remember what I said earlier: The healthiest food you can eat is the one you'll put in your mouth.

While we're on the subject of peanut butter let me share with you yet another health Nazi story to illustrate my point about seeking the "Nutrilicious." Upon seeing a jar of conventional peanut butter in my covert, yet another friend crinkled his nose and said, "Why are you eating that garbage when you could have something so much healthier, like almond butter?"

I had two thoughts at that moment. One, I needed new friends. Two, that I should at least check out his suggestion, as almonds are much healthier than peanuts. I should have stuck with thought number one. I went off to Whole Foods to dutifully buy almond butter. I took one bite of it, screwed the lid back in the jar, and tossed it into the garbage.

I'd rather eat lint off the floor.

Do not let perfection be the enemy of progress. You are on a journey to an enhanced sense of well-being not in some ghastly experiment to achieve perfection. Listen to the helpful when they point you from unhealthy to healthy. But do not listen to the health Nazis, who berate you for choosing healthy over healthiest. Whenever I'm around my health Nazi friends I do not argue with them. I do not make them wrong. I do not try to persuade them to my side of the argument.

I simply chew the Jif peanut butter with my mouth open.

It's A Party Not A Wake.

Remember, the party's in your mouth so make sure you invite partiers not mourners. If you'll allow me a short story:

> In an ancient monastery in a faraway place, a new monk arrived to join his brothers in copying books and scrolls in the monastery's scriptorium. He was assigned as a scriptor on copies of books that had already been copied by hand. One day he asked Father Florian (the Armarius of the Scriptorium), "Does not the copying by hand of other copies allow for chances of error? How do we know we are not copying the mistakes of someone else? Are they ever checked against the original?"

> Fr. Florian was set back a bit by the obvious logical observation of this youthful monk. "A very good point, my son. I will take one of the latest books down to the vault and compare it against the original."

> Fr. Florian went down to the secured vault and

began his verification. After a day had passed, the monks began to worry and went down looking for the old priest. They were sure something must have happened. As they approached the vault, they heard sobbing and crying. When they opened the door, they found Fr. Florian sobbing over the new copy and table. It was obvious to all that the poor man had been crying his heart out for a long time.

"What is the problem, Reverend Father?" asked one of the monks. "Oh, my Lord," sobbed the priest, "The word is _celebrate!_"

You are not taking a vow of culinary celibacy with The Scratch Plan. You are celebrating the experience of eating delicious foods that make you healthy and strong, even if health Nazis think you're slumming it.

Remember The Goal And You'll Get Your Results.

Our goal is to reach a high level of well-being, which requires you to honor your body's cravings for healthy _and_ unhealthy foods. This book is mostly about managing consumption of the latter, but that doesn't relieve you of the duty of getting yourself to eat and enjoy healthy foods. After all, you can't have a great sense of well-being if all you eat is empty calories, no matter how moderately you eat them. Later, I will show you how concepts designed to decrease unhealthy eating, can be used to increase your intake of healthy foods without the feeling of sacrifice.

For now, let's talk about those pesky little cravings for high fat/high carb meals that are doing you in. Like a bacon cheeseburger and a basket of fries. You tried ignoring them and they kept you up. You tried fight fighting them and they left you exhausted. You tried indulging them and they made you fat.

Clearly, you need a better way to manage them.

Where Are We?

We shifted our goal from weight loss to well-being. We are not on a diet; we are on a journey to well-being, which results in weight loss.

We avoid triggering the body's fat-promoting biological responses to dieting. We don't restrict or ban foods, set weight loss goals, or weigh ourselves constantly.

We use pain-free systematic desensitization techniques to reduce or eliminate binging. The reduction of sugar and fat enhances our sense of well-being, which results in weight loss.

We are committed to eating healthy foods. We go for the "Nutrilicious"—healthy foods that are delicious to you, even if they're mixed with not-so-healthy ingredients.

CHAPTER FOUR

How To Say No To Fat & Sugar Bombs
Without Pain Or Suffering

Learn A Delayed Gratification Technique Called
Postponement Of The Goods

Systematic desensitization works wonders on the amount of problem foods you eat, but reducing the volume is only half the equation. What about frequency? What's the point of reducing my volume to three Oreos if I end up eating that amount once or twice a day?

You can use systematic desensitization/habituation to reduce the volume of 'problem food' consumption but not the frequency of it. For that, we're going to need a different set of tools. At this point, let's expand our definition of problem foods from snacks or treats like Oreos and potato chips to 'problem meals' like a burger, fries and slaw or a plate of barbecued ribs, baked beans and mashed potatoes with gravy.

Is anyone else getting hungry?

Anyway, moderation isn't just about reducing the portion but decreasing the number of times you eat said portion.

And you're never going to be able to do that without frequently saying 'no' to problem meals you crave. But how do you deny yourself without descending into deprivation mode, which triggers the body's fat-promoting biological responses?

By using the psychological strategy of delayed gratification. Renowned psychologist Walter Mischel set off a wave of research on self-control when he published the first study on delayed gratification, which became known as The Marshmallow Test. His tests put preschoolers in a tough dilemma: Eat one marshmallow now or wait 15 minutes and have two.

The 5-year-olds sat alone in a room, facing the one marshmallow they could have immediately or the two if they waited. Mischel put a desk bell next to the treats. If the children changed their mind before the 15 minutes was up they could ring it and Mischel's assistant would enter the room and allow them to have one marshmallow. If they waited dutifully, the assistant would walk in after 15 minutes and allow them to have two.

Now, it goes without saying that self-control is one of the most important characteristics of successful living. Athletes must sacrifice their desire to relax in front of the TV and hit the fields to practice if they want to win championships. Financially astute people must resist the temptation to spend money now so they can retire comfortably. Mischel calls self-control the "master aptitude underlying emotional intelligence, essential for constructing a fulfilling life."

In fact, the ability to delay immediate gratification for a better consequence in the future is strongly associated with success later in life. Mischel proved that "high delay" children (the ones who could wait 15 minutes for two marshmallows) went on to lead much more constructive lives than "low delay" children who opted for the one marshmallow. They achieved more in their careers, they coped better with stress, and yes, they were thinner.

Which brings us to why The Scratch Plan uses a modified form of the delayed gratification technique in Mischel's Marshmallow Test. While Mischel proved that delayed gratification is a highly effective way of mastering self-control, his model has severe limitations. Recall that The Marshmallow Test offered children one marshmallow now or two fifteen minutes later. Clearly we cannot use a delayed gratification technique that says, "You can have a plate of fried chicken now or two plates of it fifteen minutes later." Our goal is to reduce the amount of food we eat, not increase it.

In trying to formulate a delayed gratification method that could work I looked at the typical ones used in the dieting world:

If I don't eat X then I'll allow myself to eat Y.

If I deprive myself of this, I'll treat myself to that.

I instinctively wanted to avoid those kinds of "If-Then" approaches because they sounded full of pain, anguish and sacrifice—the hallmarks of a diet ("If I punish myself with deprivation I'll reward myself with indulgence"). I knew it was bound to trigger my body's fight or flight response and make it biologically impossible for me to delay gratification.

As I thought about how I could construct a Marshmallow Test-inspired "If-Then plan" I knew the 'reward' for delaying a tempting food had to do two things:

1. Avoid throwing me into a diet spiral and set off my body's fight or flight syndrome.

2. Reduce or eliminate the pain of sacrificing 'now' for 'later.'

I spent a long time constructing a technique as successful and painless as desensitization was on my Oreo consumption. I kept going back to dieting's central pain point: Food restriction. Denial. Deprivation. I remember thinking, "What if I replaced deprivation with postponement? What if I replaced NO with NOT YET?

Allow me to introduce a delayed gratification technique I call *Postponement Of The Goods.* You are not going to deny yourself a problem meal; you're going to postpone its consumption to a later date when your craving for it is at a higher level.

Wait, what does that mean?

Well, think about your favorite problem meal. Maybe a stack of pancakes dripping with butter, maple syrup and three strips of bacon? (SQUIRREL!).

You are not going to deny yourself a problem meal; you're going to postpone its consumption until your craving for it gets stronger.

Now be honest—is the intensity for those pancakes always banging the craving meter at a '10'? Of course not. It fluctuates in a spectrum between 1 (low) and 10 (you'd knock your grandmother over to lick the syrup). The idea for *Postponement Of The Goods* is to:

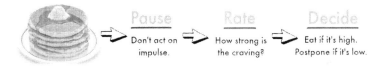

Pause — Don't act on impulse. → Rate — How strong is the craving? → Decide — Eat if it's high. Postpone if it's low.

Pause. Rate. Decide. This is your three word mantra before you reach for any kind of food. When it comes to eating you have to navigate between two minefields: Triggering the fight or flight response (caused by deprivation, rigid scheduling of foods or having a rewards concept attached to them) and triggering weight gain from unrestricted eating. *Postponement Of The Goods* helps you sail smoothly between the two with a simple framework to guide your decision:

1. **Pause.** Take stock of the situation.

2. **Rate.** On a scale of 1 to 10, how would you rank your craving?

3. **Decide.** Base it on a pre-agreed intensity level that triggers a decision to eat the food. For the sake of argument, let's say it's a "7."

Let's see how this plays out…

> **If:** The craving intensity is seven or higher…
> **Then:** Eat the food now.

> **If:** The craving intensity is six or lower…
> **Then:** Postpone until the intensity is higher.

Notice that your options are not "eat" or "don't eat." They're "eat" or "postpone." I'm not quibbling with semantics here. The body responds much better to LATER than to NO. No means you're on a diet. Later means you're waiting for a better time to enjoy the food.

Earn Your Body's Trust.

Trust is a key factor in convincing your body not to trigger its fat inducing biological responses to deprivation. You must be authentic about it. If you postpone eating the food because the craving intensity didn't meet your criteria, then you MUST eat the food when it does. Otherwise your body will see right through the manipulation and associate LATER with LIAR and go into fight or flight response.

Dr. Mischel understood the importance of trust in getting his subjects to participate. His assistants would play with the children before the start of the experiment to establish comfort. Then they'd sit the child at a table with a desk bell. For 'practice,' the assistants would repeatedly step out of the room and rush in immediately when the child rang the bell. They'd say something like "See? I came back!" They proved to the child that if they rang the bell after waiting 15 minutes the assistants would rush in and feed them the two marshmallows.

Think of your body as the child in The Marshmallow Test. You have to earn its trust by keeping your promise. Imagine what kind of results Mischel would have gotten if the children doubted that delaying gratification would result in getting 2 marshmallows.

Mischel kept his word to the children; you keep yours to your body. If the intensity of your craving for a problem meal hits a pre-agreed trigger, then you need to indulge. Every time. Not sometimes. Always.

Why Pause-Rate-Decide Works.

Postponement of the Goods works because it spaces out the eating of problematic foods without unduly stressing the body. It teaches you discipline without suffering. There is not much pain in denying yourself a plate of spaghetti and meatballs (with lots of garlic bread!) when you *kind of* want it as opposed to when you *really* want it. This skill—letting the intensity level of your cravings determine when you will eat high fat/high calorie foods—will, over time dramatically improve your ability to lose weight without going on a diet.

Now, I want you to notice a couple of things about *Postponement of the Goods*. This is not a plan about resisting temptation; it's about yielding to it <u>if</u> the craving intensity meets your criteria. And the reward isn't more food; it's a better experience of it.

Think about that. Are you more likely to enjoy a plate of spaghetti and meatballs (with lots of garlic bread!) when your craving is at a '2' or a '10'?

At '2' it's good, not great. At '10' it's great, not good. You will better appreciate the aroma, taste more of the flavors, and lose yourself in the experience. You want a better experience of food? Pause. Rate. Decide.

How Will It Help You Lose Weight?

You know I hate that question because weight loss is not our goal, but the concern is valid so let me address it.

> Notice that your options are not "eat" or "don't eat." They're "eat" or "postpone."

It's a fact that most of us eat problem foods with no or low-cravings, at least part of the time. I'm not talking about 'distracted' eating, like emptying a bag of pretzels while you watch TV. I mean eating when you're simply not that hungry or hungry, but not necessarily for the food you're eating. Have you ever finished eating a bunch of ice cream and thought, "That was delicious but why did I eat it? I didn't want it that badly." *That's* what I call low or no-craving eating.

And that's what *Postponement of the Goods* cuts out—eating when you have no/low cravings. You're going to be amazed at how many problem foods you eat with a low intensity craving—and how many you can cut out by simply postponing their intake until the craving intensity reaches the trigger mark. All you have to do is Pause. Rate. Decide.

How many carbs, fat, calories (or whatever you like to count) do you think you'd cut out if you only ate problem foods when your craving reached a '7' or higher? Let's take a look at one possible scenario. Let's say that you, like your fellow Americans, eat an average of 63 donuts a year (Source:

Baltimore Sun). If we plotted out your annual donut consumption according to the craving level you had for it at the time of consumption, it might look something like this:

Your Annual Donut Consumption

How Painful Is Your Craving?

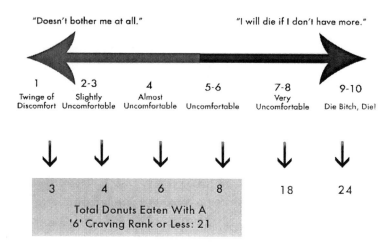

"Doesn't bother me at all."

"I will die if I don't have more."

1	2-3	4	5-6	7-8	9-10
Twinge of Discomfort	Slightly Uncomfortable	Almost Uncomfortable	Uncomfortable	Very Uncomfortable	Die Bitch, Die!

| 3 | 4 | 6 | 8 | 18 | 24 |

Total Donuts Eaten With A
'6' Craving Rank or Less: 21

Do The Math.

Let's pretend you ate 63 Krispy Kreme glazed donuts over the course of a year. Each donut contains 200 calories, 12 grams of fat, and 10 grams of sugars. Multiply that against the 21 donuts you ate when your craving was '6' or below and they represent:

- 4,200 calories

- 252 grams of fat

- 210 grams of sugar

Postponement Of The Goods could have saved you the trouble of ingesting 21 fat bombs at little or no distress to you. Now, this may not sound like a lot—after all 4,200 calories over the course of a year is only about 80 calories a week. But you're going to be using *Postponement Of The Goods* for <u>every single problem food or meal in your diet.</u> Now you're looking at a very significant reduction in calories, fat and sugars. And all you have to do is Pause. Rate. Decide.

What's The Right Intensity Trigger For You?

I have no idea. It's your decision. Everybody is different. Mine is '7' because that's the start of real pain. *For me.* You might have a lower trigger point. If even light cravings tend to derail you then knock your trigger back to '4', '5' or '6.' The number doesn't matter. That you have a number does. I use a '7.' I have friends that use a '5.' If you have to start with a '3', so what? You can ratchet up as time goes on.

Be aware that your inner dieter will try to game the system by choosing a painful trigger level (like a '9') because it thinks it will lose weight faster. The thing is, you *will* lose weight faster if you choose '9'. But then you'll set off your body's fight or flight system, get ravenously hungry and slow down your metabolism. The wheels will come off the desert cart, if you will, and you're right back to the dieter's dilemma: Try, fail, shame. Try, fail, despair. Try, fail, panic.

Choose the trigger honestly by asking yourself two questions:

The reward for "postponing the goods" isn't more food; it's a better experience of it.

1. "How badly do I want this food?"

If you want it badly enough you should have it. Suffering is never an option. But how do you *know* if you want it badly? This is what happens to me: I start obsessing about the food. I can't get the thought of how it would taste out of my mind. I vividly picture the color, texture and smell. I mutter things like "Get in my belly!"

2. "Would I experience real pain if I deny myself this meal?"

Again, the point is to *avoid* suffering. Here are the pain markers I look for: I start getting upset at the thought of not having it. I start rationalizing why I should have it ("I've been eating good all week—I deserve it!"). I get angry with myself for having thoughts of passing it up. I start remembering how empty and frustrated I felt the last time I didn't have this food when I really wanted it.

How I Established '7' As My Trigger Point.

Look at the two questions above and how I answered them. '7' is the *beginning point* of all those thoughts and feelings. Do not make the mistake of establishing your trigger point at a mid or end-point. Our goal is to postpone consumption of the goods with so little pain that it is eminently manageable.

Setting a trigger point is highly subjective because pain, while real, is defined by your opinion of it, not somebody else's. I don't wait for a headache to fully blossom before taking an aspirin. I do it at the first sign I'm getting one. Set your trigger point at the first signs of a painful craving.

Keep Your Eye On The Donut And Not On The Hole.

Let's say a coworker plunks down a box of Krispy Kreme doughnuts on the conference room table. Somebody opens the lid of the box and the sweet smell of baked sugar fills the room, making half the people in the room act like dogs trying to get out of a car that just pulled up to a park. Everyone reaches in and grabs their gift from the gods. Do you automatically reach for the yeasty goodness? Here's how I use the *Postponement Of The Goods* technique in this scenario:

Scenario One

Pause: How badly do I want this doughnut on a scale of 1-10?

Rate: 5

Decide: I don't eat the doughnut. I'm careful to think—and sometimes say out loud—"I'll have a doughnut when my craving for it hits a 7 or higher."

Discussion: It is not painful to avoid a delicious food when the urge for it exists but doesn't dominate. Yes, it's somewhat uncomfortable but completely manageable. My body doesn't rebel because it knows unequivocally that I mean what I say. If a craving for a Krispy Kreme glazed donut ranks seven or higher I always indulge. ALWAYS. Not "often," not "sometimes." ALWAYS.

And I don't do it grudgingly. I don't make myself feel guilty. I serve myself donuts *gleefully*. My body trusts my decisions 100% because I have never tried to manipulate it, take back my word or fool it into doing what I want. I have taught my body a critical lesson:

No Never Means No.
It Means Not Now.

Why Does Postponement Work?

Think of it this way. Have you ever wanted to be intimate with a partner who wasn't in the mood? You bust a move and he or she squirms away. You try to kiss them on the lips and they give you a cheek. You put your arm around them and they fling it away. You are rebuffed at every front (or back depending on your preferences). Finally, your partner turns to you and sneers, "What part of no do you not understand!?"

How do you feel? Unloved. Unwanted. Neglected. Frustrated. Angry. And if it happens often enough, you start doubting the relationship will survive.

Now let me propose a different scenario. You want to be intimate. You bust a move and he or she squirms away. You try a kiss on the lips and they give you a cheek. You put your arm around them but they don't fling it away. Instead, they gently take your hand in theirs and say, "Honey, not tonight. How about tomorrow night?"

How do you feel? Disappointed but hopeful.

Contrast that to how you felt in the earlier scenario—unloved, unwanted, neglected, frustrated and angry. Rejection inflicts terrible damage. Postponement does not. And that is at the heart of my *Postponement of the Goods* technique: Don't reject; postpone. Your body will not go into fight or flight when it is disappointed but hopeful. It absolutely will go into fat-promoting biological responses when it feels abandoned, neglected, and doubtful of its survival. Whether it's in the kitchen or the bedroom a postponement is easier to take than a rejection.

Scenario Two

Pause: How badly do I want this doughnut on a scale of 1-10?

Rate: 8

Decide: I eat it. Maybe two. Possibly three.

Discussion: Promises, promises. It's important to keep them. I will say to myself, "See? Look how much more I get to enjoy the doughnut at a 8 ranking than if I had eaten it at a 5 ranking." I make it a point to remind myself that there is little pain and real joy to keeping my word.

In some ways *Postponement Of The Goods* isn't a delayed gratification technique so much as an immediate gratification plan moderated by the intensity of the craving. It acknowledges that exercising restraint only works if you don't set off the body's fight or flight response. In that sense, it pairs self-control with self-realization.

Postponement of the Goods hews closely to Mischel's understanding of self-control. First, it uses an if-then plan: "*If* my craving is a seven or higher *then* I will eat the doughnut." This buys you a few seconds to consider your options as opposed to blindly following your body's desire for immediate gratification.

Second, it offers the benefit of delayed gratification: A better outcome if you wait. Mischel's study asked children what would be more pleasurable—one or 2 marshmallows? *Postponement of the Goods* asks adults a similar question: What would be more pleasurable—eating marshmallows when your craving is high or low? Pause. Rate. Decide.

> **No Never Means No.
> It Means Not Now.**

What If You Can't Identify The Intensity Level Of Your Craving?

It's easy to talk about cravings when they're banging the desire meter to the right and setting off five-alarm bells and bongs because they're so urgent. But not all cravings are that dramatic and if you're not used to "rating the craving" you may feel a little lost and confused.

Earlier I showed you a craving status bar that ranked the intensity from a low of 1 to a high of 10. Assigning an accurate number may be hard at first (it was for me). After all, most of us have never stopped to ask ourselves, "How much do I want this food?" We simply ate it at the merest flicker of desire.

If you're having trouble assigning a number you might want to use a "High, Medium, or Low" scale. For example, something like this:

How Badly Do You Want This Food?

High

- You're obsessing about it.
- You're not entertaining other options.
- You get upset at the thought of not having it.

Medium

- You want it, but it's not a 'must have'.
- It's the leading option, but you're considering others.
- You'd be disappointed, but not upset, if you didn't get it.

Low

- You kinda/sorta want it.
- You're considering other options.
- You'd be mildy disappointed if you didn't get it.

It is imperative to use some way of marking the intensity of the food you're considering eating because it gives you the chance to avoid impulsive, no/low craving eating. From here on out you should never put anything in your mouth without first knowing how badly you want it. This is mindful eating. In the split second it takes to become aware of the craving intensity you're at choice, not habit.

The good thing about marking craving intensities is that it's easy, fun and takes about five seconds. You don't need to write anything down, you don't need to study anything. Hell, you don't even need to get it right. "About right" will do. You're not pitching toward perfection; you're aiming for mindfulness.

The best part is that it doesn't take very long for the Pause-Rate-Decide mindfulness technique to become automatic. I've internalized it so deeply that it is no longer a process but a mindset. I don't actually stop to ask myself how badly I want a particular food anymore—just like you don't actually stop to ask yourself what to do when a traffic light turns green. You just *know*.

> It isn't about resisting temptation; it's about yielding to it—when your craving hits the trigger mark.

What if it takes you longer to internalize the process because you keep forgetting to rate your cravings? Well, that would make you human, wouldn't it? Don't worry about it. You're not in a race and you're not on a diet. You're going to be doing this for the rest of your life, so what's a few forgets? Gently remind yourself to do it next time. Remember, the process is not a burden; it's simply a question: "How badly do I want this food?" So here, relax, have another cookie.

Just remember to ask yourself how badly you want it.

Postponing The Goods will help you significantly reduce no/ low craving or mindless eating and binging. Think about it —how often do we eat because we're supposed to, not necessarily because we want to? Noon *is* lunchtime, whether you're hungry or not. We also tend to eat what's in front of us or what's available (because we have the opportunity— even gas stations have food). We also tend to veg out and eat mindlessly out of bags or simply because somebody offered us food. In each of these cases rating your cravings gives you the opportunity to exercise choice; something that is probably lacking in your eating habits right now.

What If You Forget To Rate The Crave?

Scenario: Somebody left a plate of "Everything" bagels in the office lunchroom with a note: "Enjoy!"

Pause: You don't. You forgot! Instead, you act on impulse. You grab it and growl, spreading cream cheese and good will everywhere.

Rate: You don't. You forgot! As soon as you take the last bite you remember the bit about rating the craving.

Decide: Now what?

Discussion: What should your penance be? None. You're not on a diet and we don't operate on the basis of punishment and reward. We operate on maximizing wellness.

If you forget to rate the crave before you cave, do it afterwards. Think back. How badly did you want the bagel *before* the first bite? Assign a number (1-10) or a temperature (low, medium or high). If it reached your craving trigger point ('7' or 'high') then congratulations—you were right for eating the bagel.

But if it didn't and you find yourself saying, "I wasn't that hungry—why did I eat that bagel?" then remember that icky feeling the next time you're faced with temptation. It'll remind you to rank your desire before you start chomping away.

Avoid Regret By Rating The Craving.

Say Goodbye To Will Power Fatigue.

All delayed gratification techniques require some exercise of will power, which is often experienced as a limited, easily depleted resource. Like a bank account, the more you use it the less you've got. But that's only true if exercising will power means enduring sharp, prolonged pain. Dieting is the best example of that. Who among us can cope with constant deprivation?

Fortunately, you will never experience will power fatigue with *Postponing the Goods* because you will never experience unendurable pain. Remember, *Postponing the Goods* isn't about resisting temptation; it's about yielding to it. And it's always at the moment you reach your pain threshold (the trigger point). Experiencing too much pain at a '7'? Then lower your trigger point to a 5 or 6. You will not suffer. Ever.

In The Marshmallow Test, children came up with coping strategies to ease the pain—by turning away from the marshmallow, distracting themselves (singing, playing) or desperately trying to think of something else. The Marshmallow Test asked children to suffer. *Postponing The Goods* asks no such thing.

In dieting, will power comes down to how much pain you can take. In the journey to well-being will power is about how much of it you can avoid. The Scratch Plan isn't about deprivation; it's about indulgence. It's about joyfully, artfully self-regulating so that you can eat what you want without throwing your body into mayday mayhem. You will never experience will power fatigue because there is nothing to be fatigued about. It's a three-step, five-second, pain-free process: Pause. Rate. Decide.

What If You Have Problems With Impulse Control?

You're at a Super Bowl party and somebody wheels out a big, thick Sicilian pizza. The crowd oohs and aaahs. You dutifully Pause, Rate and Decide. You give it a '4'—way below your '7' trigger point, but you take a slice anyway. Two, actually. What's going on?

You ate the pizza even though it was considerably below your stated pain threshold. This happened a lot to me when I first started—I often chose to eat a food even though the craving wasn't very strong. I would Pause, Rate and Decide …against my pre-agreed trigger point.

Typically, it occurred when internal or environmental factors didn't go my way. For instance, if I was starving and the hunger overwhelmed my mindfulness. Or if I was nervous or anxious and ate to calm or comfort myself. Or if I didn't want to insult the host at a private dinner. Or if I wanted to join the fun of communal eating.

> Build your body's trust so it knows you are not rejecting the now as much as postponing for later.

The world is a machination against mindfulness, a connivance against mastery and a scheme against self-control. But that's okay because we're aiming for progress not perfection. There will be times that internal or environmental situations will overwhelm your ability to Pause-Rate-Decide properly. It's important to audit your thoughts when this happens. Are you blaming yourself? Feeling guilty? That's diet-think.

Here's a better way: Reframe your actions from right/wrong to helpful/unhelpful. Was your decision 'wrong' or unhelpful? There is a lot of baggage attached to the former and none to the latter.

Making a decision to eat a food three or four points below your trigger level is not a moral failure. It is an understandable reaction to internal or external pressure. Do not forgive yourself, gather your strength and promise to do better next time. A decision a few degrees off the mark does not require forgiveness.

You do not need to marshal your resources because the Pause-Rate-Decide process does not ask you to white knuckle your way through a painful craving. It asks you to *avoid* pain by deciding affirmatively in the presence of a strong craving.

And you do not need to do better next time because you have the rest of your life to make better decisions. In the context of making tens of thousands of eating decisions in the next 20, 30, 40 or 50 years, your next decision isn't going to ruin anything.

So give yourself a break. This is a long and winding road—occasional potholes are to be expected. A few unhelpful decisions aren't going to matter. Now, if you find yourself constantly and consistently having problems with impulse control there are a couple of things that will help.

Impulse Or Mindfulness? Regret Or Rejoice?

The first is to formalize your attention on the future. All delayed gratification techniques can be boiled down to one central conflict: Now vs. Later. It will be easier to make a helpful decision if you turn your attention away from Now and focus on Later.

Delayed gratification studies show that people are much more likely to delay pleasure if they have a firm grasp of what the delay buys them. For example, cigarette smokers who focus on the long-term consequences of cigarette smoking (lung cancer) significantly increase their ability to stay away from cigarettes. All respects to Buddhism and Zen, "staying in the now" is a terrible place to be if you want to master self-control. Tomorrow is a much better place than today.

It's easy to see the benefits of Later to a cigarette smoker—a cancer free life. But what are the benefits of impulse control over food to you? Raise your hand if you said, "Losing weight." Now slap yourself with that hand. You are not on a diet. You're on a journey toward well-being. I don't want you to concentrate on the possibility of thinness; I want you to concentrate on the certainty of pleasure.

Being on a diet forces you to think about weight. Being on a journey toward well-being invites you to think about health and pleasure. A dieter shifts her perspective from Now to Later by concentrating on how thin her waistline will get. The traveler to well-being shifts it by concentrating on how much more pleasure she's going to get out of food. Again, eating a bowl of spaghetti and meatballs (with garlic bread!) is a lot more pleasurable at a '10' than a '2.'

How does the focus on pleasure help delay gratification? Let's go back to that Super Bowl party and the Sicilian pizza. Let's say you gave your craving a four rating (relatively low) but you can sense that you're about to give in to impulse. Concentrate on how much more pleasure you're going to get out of that pizza when the craving hits a seven, eight, nine or ten.

You can cut out a third to two thirds of your problem foods not by deprivation but by postponement.

Contrast how you felt the last time you ate a pizza with a

low craving to the last time you ate a pizza with a high craving. Notice how much more flavorful the pizza was at the high craving. Remember how satisfied you felt? Amp up the desire to experience that level of satisfaction again. Ask yourself, *"Am I willing to put off a mediocre experience now for an intense one later?"*

If the answer is no, then eat the pizza without guilt. You have tens of thousands of decisions to make in the future—this one is not going to matter. If the answer is yes—you <u>are</u> willing to delay "mediocre now" for "intense later"—then it's critical that you get yourself over to a pizza joint the minute you have a strong craving for one. Build your body's trust so it knows you are not rejecting the now as much as postponing for later.

The Secret To Mastering Self-Control: Psychological Distancing

The second way to put some order around impulse control is something called "psychological distancing." In The Marshmallow Test Walter Mischel noticed that children who could delay gratification would often distance themselves from the marshmallow in front of them by turning it into an abstraction. For example, they would imagine it as framed and hanging on the wall. Why? Because, as one child memorably stated, "You can't eat a picture!"

Mischel was so impressed by the power of psychological distancing to build "high delay" skills he went on to study the phenomenon further. He soon discovered new ways to help people "self-distance" from painful experiences like social rejection and heartbreak. In an especially clever study he split people who had experienced overwhelmingly negative feelings from a breakup into two groups. Half were asked to reflect on the breakup from their own perspective and try to understand their feelings (the way we normally process experiences).

But he asked the other half to "visualize the experience from the perspective of a fly on the wall." In other words, to psychologically distance themselves from their own perspectives. The results were dramatic. The self-immersion group that reflected from their point of view became more emotional, more agitated and increased their anguish as they relived the breakup. But the self-distanced group showed much less emotions, used more abstract terms to describe their feelings and experienced more emotional stability. Mischel proved that seeing things from your own perspective tends to recount and reactivate negative feelings while distancing yourself helps reappraise them.

What does all this have to do with food? The next time you run into problems with Sicilian pizza pretend you're a fly on the wall or a narrator in a movie and view the perspective from there. Oh, and don't forget to frame the pizza and hang it on a wall. You can't eat a picture!

Weight Loss vs. Well-being.

I want to stress an important point here. You are not punishing yourself when you say no to a food with a 6 or below craving. And neither are you rewarding yourself when you say yes to a food with a seven or higher craving. That is the mentality of a dieter and we are not on a diet. When you say no to a '6' or below or yes to a '7' or higher you are enhancing your well-being. *Postponement of the Goods* maximizes the pleasure you take out of food. And pleasure is a hallmark of well-being.

Postponement of the Goods also adds to well-being by assuring you of a healthier diet. As time goes on you will see that *Postponement of the Goods* cuts out a lot of sugar, salt, fat and calories from your diet. It has no choice but to because you will be saying "no" to those doughnuts (or any problem food or meal) many, many times for the rest of your life. This is simply because many of your cravings will not rise to your trigger point, not because you're on a diet.

> Ask yourself, "Am I willing to put off a mediocre experience now for an intense one later?"

Right now I'm betting that you don't make a distinction between low, medium and high levels of cravings for problem foods. I'm guessing you pretty much eat them as long as there is an iota of desire. *Postponement of the Goods* forces you to assess the craving before you proceed with a simple formula: Pause. Rate. Decide.

Since you will only indulge with a craving of say, a seven or higher, you are going to cut out a significant portion of your current indulgences. I know I cut mine by one third to two thirds, depending on the food. Think about that for a moment: you can cut out a third to two thirds of your problem foods not by deprivation but by postponement.

So let's review. *Postponement of the Goods* enhances the pleasure you take out a food and minimizes the frequency of consuming problem foods, which enhances your overall health. Does that sound like a diet to you? It shouldn't. Yet it results in weight loss. No, it will not happen right away. And no, it won't even happen in the first couple of months. But over time, as you get better and better at postponing the goods, you will see how indispensable it is to the results you're seeking.

How To Manage Emotions Around Not Losing Weight Quickly.

There are basically two ways to get to the top of a mountain —*directly* towards the top or *indirectly* through switchbacks that ring the sides of the mountain.

When the mountain is 'simple' (gentle slope, no cliffs) you can use the direct method and literally walk straight to the top in a straight line. But most mountains aren't simple and unless you're willing to risk your life with ropes, harnesses, crampons, carabiners, ice axes, and pulleys, you are much better off going the longer way—through the switchbacks.

Don't get discouraged with The Scratch Plan just because you can't see the top of Weight Loss Mountain. How many times have you climbed a peak using switchbacks that hid the top from view for long stretches? How many times have they temporarily taken you *down* the mountain not up? You didn't panic because you knew the trail was bypassing major obstacles (boulders, waterfalls) that temporarily forced you to lose altitude. You knew that it was just a matter of time before the trail gained elevation on its way to the top.

Delayed gratification techniques like *Postponement Of The Goods* and the one I'm about to introduce are like trails that sometimes go down before they up. They are not going help you lose weight quickly. In fact, they may temporarily make you gain weight, just as some parts of a trail temporarily make you lose altitude in order to bypass obstacles. And just so we're clear, the obstacles we're trying to get around are the body's fat-promoting biological responses to dieting.

Now, I want to introduce you to another devilish delayed gratification technique guaranteed to minimize or eliminate all those low-rent foods you're eating. You know, like grocery store sheet cakes.

Isn't it time you upgraded to higher quality crap?

Where Are We?

We shifted our goal from weight loss to well-being. We are not on a diet; we are on a journey to well-being.

We avoid triggering the body's fat-promoting biological responses to dieting. We don't restrict or ban foods, set weight loss goals, or weigh ourselves constantly.

We use pain-free systematic desensitization techniques to reduce or eliminate binging. The reduction of sugar and fat enhances our sense of well-being, which results in weight loss.

We are committed to eating healthy foods. We go for the "Nutrilicious"—healthy foods that are delicious to you, even if they're mixed with not-so-healthy ingredients.

We use a delayed gratification technique called *Postponement Of The Goods* to reduce the frequency with which we eat problem foods. We know that "No" never means no. It means later.

We shifted our goal from weight loss to well-being. We are not on a diet; we are on a journey to well-being.

We avoid triggering the body's fat-promoting biological responses to dieting. We don't restrict or ban foods, set weight loss goals, or weigh ourselves constantly.

We use pain-free systematic desensitization techniques to reduce or eliminate binging. The reduction of sugar and fat enhances our sense of well-being, which results in weight loss.

We are committed to eating healthy foods. We go for the "Nutrilicious"—healthy foods that are delicious to you, even if they're mixed with not-so-healthy ingredients.

We use a delayed gratification technique called *Postponement Of The Goods* to reduce the frequency with which we eat problem foods. We know that "No" never means no. It means later.

CHAPTER FIVE

How To Stop Eating Junk Food and Other High Calorie/High Sugar Foods

Learn a delayed gratification technique called Bargaining For Higher Quality Crap

The Marshmallow Test inspired me to develop a second delayed gratification technique but instead of basing it on quantity ("one marshmallow now or two later") I based it on quality ("low quality crap now or higher quality crap later").

First, some background. A lot of us eat tasty but crappy food. A great example is fast food—lots of salt, sugar, low quality ingredients, preservatives and the like. Don't get me wrong, some of it is delicious. Take the McGriddle from McDonald's. It's a breakfast sandwich with bacon, egg and cheese between two maple-flavored-pancakes. It's proof that God exists.

Still, it's crap. Tasty, but crap. While tasty aligns with our goal of enhanced well-being, crap does not. A dieter's solution would be to either cut out the McGriddle altogether or reconstruct it with fake cheese, egg whites, bacon-flavored tofu, and gluten-free bread. Let me tell you something: I only speak English but I know how to say "Kill me now" in eight different languages.

If the dieter's solution is to deprive or deform what is the well-being solution? If I ask you to delay the gratification of eating a McGriddle what do you get in return for waiting? Two McGriddles? Of course not.

How about something better than a McGriddle? How about a breakfast sandwich made out of organic eggs, real cheese and apple-wood smoked bacon on fresh-baked ciabatta? I don't care how good the McGriddle is, it can't compare to what I just described. I'm not sure there's much of a difference in salt, sugar or fat content but there are no preservatives, the ingredients are of much higher quality and the taste, Oh, my God, the taste! (scrunches fingers together, touches lips and blows out a kiss).

Allow me to introduce a delayed gratification technique I call *Bargaining for Higher-Quality Crap*. It's based on a simple notion: Say no to crap now so you can have higher-quality crap later. Or as Professor Mischel might have put it to the preschoolers: "Say no to the store-bought marshmallow now so you can have a fresh baked cookie later."

Mischel's delayed gratification experiment rewarded children with volume (more marshmallows). Mine rewards you with quality (a tastier experience). Here's how it works:

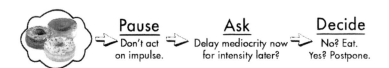

Pause Don't act on impulse. **Ask** Delay mediocrity now for intensity later? **Decide** No? Eat. Yes? Postpone.

Pause. Ask. Decide. This is your second three-word mantra you need to repeat before you put anything in your mouth. Let's talk about why *Bargaining for Higher-Quality Crap* is such an important part of our strategy. What we're doing is setting a higher threshold for quality. The higher the quality the more pleasure you will get out of food. Pleasure as I've stated again and again, is an important aspect of well-being. So is health. When you replace low-quality ingredients with high-quality ingredients you will improve your health, which improves your sense of well-being. Holding out for higher-quality crap decreases the chances that you're going to eat things that will do harm to your body.

Pleasure and health helps move us from the vicious cycle of dieting to the virtuous circle of well-being. So don't settle for crap even in junk food. If you're going to eat a high carb/high fat snack or meal then by God, make it the highest quality, best possible tasting high fat/high carb food.

I love desserts. Cakes, cookies, pies, ice cream. You name it I eat it (when my craving intensity reaches 7+ of course), but I've learned over time to bargain for higher quality crap. I don't eat low-rent stuff like a grocery store sheet cake at a birthday party. It's no to boxed coffee cake but if I run into a homemade cinnamon roll? I'm on it like frosting on a Cinnabon.

The idea is to train your body to like better quality foods even if they are fat and sugar bombs. My body never goes into fight or flight response because I am authentic about

Don't deny yourself foods you crave; postpone eating them until you can find a higher quality version of them.

the trade-off. I don't deny myself foods I crave; I postpone eating them until I can find a higher quality version of them. Pause-Ask-Decide has the happy consequence of reducing the amount of fat bombs I eat. Low-quality tripe is cheap and it's everywhere; high-quality crap is more expensive and harder to find. These two facts reduce the chances of finding fat bombs worthy of eating.

Bargaining For Higher Quality Crap is very similar to *Postponement Of The Goods*. They're both delayed gratification techniques that use the concept of postponement rather than deprivation. And they both deliver more pleasure if you agree to the delay. It's just that one uses craving intensity as a trigger to eat while the other uses a quality consideration.

It's important not to see either of these delayed gratification techniques as a system of rewards for "being good." That's diet-think. Instead, see it as a system for putting more health and pleasure into your life.

For example, I consider *Bargaining For Higher Quality Crap* as something that my body deserves, not because it's being "good" but because it runs better when I give it higher quality food. You would never think of serving your child higher quality food because she was on good behavior. You do it whether she misbehaved or not. You serve her higher quality food because you love her unconditionally and know that her body and mind will be better for it. The same concept applies here: Hold out for high quality food not as a reward, but as a way of showing unconditional love to yourself.

Delicious, high quality food is not the reward for trying to be thin; it's the reward for being human.

Ask.	"Am I willing to hold off eating this now for something better later?"
Decide.	There will be times you'll be willing to delay and times you won't. You will not punish yourself if you don't delay nor praise yourself if you do. You will simply keep moving toward higher-quality crap at your own pace.
	~~cancer gods are looking at you and whis~~ pering, "I saw him first; he's mine!"

Discussion: If you don't Pause-Ask-Decide you are acting out of impulse rather than mindfulness. If you do, you're at choice not habit. Mindfulness and impulsiveness often reach the same conclusion ("I'll take it!") but they come at it from different perspectives. Impulsiveness always results in the same decision; mindfulness does not. One victimizes, the other empowers.

Now, how can deciding to eat the sheet cake empower you? Because it was a mindful decision rather than an impulsive reaction. And once you start making mindful decisions all the time you'll find yourself postponing for higher quality more and more.

Instead of feeling guilty that you ate the cake (that's diet-think) ask yourself two simple questions: How tasty was the cake and how good do you feel after eating it? Are you satisfied? Gratified? If the cake was tasty and satisfying then maybe you should never bargain for higher quality when it comes to sheet cake. Maybe part of your journey to well-being includes crappy sheet cake. Hell, mine includes Oreos —why shouldn't yours include store-bought goodies, too?

But if the cake wasn't tasty or satisfying then use that experience to inform your next decision. Upon facing a temptation I often say to myself, "Remember the last time you ate a couple of boxed donuts from the gas station? You could taste the chemicals. Let's skip it this time and get some fresh ones at Dunkin' Donuts in a few days."

Use yesterday's negative experiences to form tomorrow's positive outcomes.

In a situation like this a little self-talk goes a long way. Something on the order of, "I promise that if I skip this sheet cake I'll have Aunt Edna's homemade red velvet cake. Think how much better it'll taste than this garbage!" If you have any doubt about how much better Aunt Edna's homemade red velvet cake tastes than a Wal-Mart sheet cake I invite you to do a side-by-side taste test. Earlier I said that the party's in your mouth so don't invite boring guests. A grocery store sheet cake is a snoozer guest who'll put the dog to sleep. Aunt Edna's cake is a party favor that'll have your boss dancing with a lampshade on his head.

Go for the lampshade.

Now, what happens if you won't see Aunt Edna for months and months? The truth is that you need to indulge in a higher-quality alternative sooner than later. The longer you go between denying yourself lower-quality crap and eating its higher-quality cousin the likelier this delayed gratification technique will fail. It won't be long before your body recognizes that you're trying to trick it into a diet and it will trigger its fat-promoting responses (making you hungrier and slowing down your metabolism).

Keeping your word is an important aspect of mindfulness. You will not be able to *consistently* get your body to forgo a cheapo sheet cake if you are inconsistent about delivering a higher-quality alternative. "Delayed gratification" means exactly that—you are delaying gratification, not eliminating it.

As you first practice *Bargaining For Higher Quality Crap*, be sure to actually seek out a higher-quality alternative within the next 24 to 48 hours. As you get better at this and as your body trusts your decisions to delay more and more you'll be able to go longer and longer between indulgences.

Bottom line: Pay Aunt Edna a visit soon or darken the door of your nearest bakery.

How Long Will It Take To Internalize Bargaining For Higher Quality Crap?

Fortunately, like *Postponing the Goods*, it doesn't require much effort. There's no homework, no preparation, and the decision to delay or not takes about five seconds. Getting good at it isn't about working hard as much as it is simply remembering the three-step, five-second process: Pause. Ask. Decide. The question is simple. "Am I willing to postpone eating this today for something better tomorrow?"

Essentially, you are building a habit and habits take time to build. Don't beat yourself up because you ate the grocery store cake. There's nothing wrong with eating it. You are not on a diet. You simply chose not to postpone for a higher-quality alternative.

How To Handle The Emotional Fallout Of NOT Postponing.

No matter how many times I say it I know that you are going to lapse into diet-think and consider NOT postponing for a higher-quality alternative as an abysmal failure. Gently remind yourself that you're not on a diet; you're on a journey toward well-being. The fact that you *decided* not to postpone is a huge sign of progress because earlier it would not even have occurred to you that postponement was an option. Congratulate yourself for arriving at choice and not staying stuck on impulse.

By the way, your goal isn't to *always* postpone; it is to *often* postpone. In that scenario there is no success or failure, just an emotion-free decision. Once you start postponing—<u>often but not always</u>—the virtuous circle of well-being takes over and you'll find yourself unconsciously postponing so much that you'll come close to cutting out all low-quality crap. Your body will get so much pleasure out of the higher-quality goods it will start craving them. And at that point postponement isn't just easy; it's automatic.

> The question is simple. "Am I willing to postpone eating this now for something better later?"

Let's talk about 'failing' for a moment. Like learning any new habit, *Bargaining For Higher Quality Crap* takes practice. I 'failed' a LOT when I started. I often ate crappy stuff even after I offered myself a better version of it. But every 'failure' helped shape my later successes by paving the way to more consistently satisfying decisions.

For example, I remembered how disappointing it was to crave for cream in my coffee and pour milk instead. I didn't want to have those experiences again so I made decisions that gave me better ones. My point is that you can look at a decision that led to an unsatisfying experience as a 'failure' or as a vivid reminder to make better decisions.

If you're wondering why I put quotes around 'fail' it's because I have a different definition of it than you do. If I decided to eat sheet cake you'd probably think I 'failed' because I broke my word, "gave in" or because I ate a verboten food that'll eventually make me fat. But only a dieter would think that way. A diet is a promise you break. A journey to well-being is a direction you take. No journey is a straight line—they're filled with all kinds of curves and angles. Is it a 'failure' if the journey temporarily takes you east-ish rather than east? What difference does it make as long as you're headed in the right direction?

And don't get me started on verboten foods. There is no such thing as a food you can't or shouldn't have in your journey to well-being. There is only how much and how frequently you can have them. No, 'failure' isn't about breaking your word, "giving in" or eating fattening food. The real 'failure' is the deeply unsatisfying feeling of appeasing an urgent craving with mediocre food.

Have you ever had a '10' craving for ice cream and eaten a cheap brand that wasn't creamy and tasted chalky? *Deeply unsatisfying.* Ever jones for chocolate chip cookies and indulged it with brittle little brats that skimped on the chocolate? *Immensely disappointing.* Ever slake your thirst for a deep-bodied Bordeaux with watered-down Kool-Aid? *Incredibly disappointing.* No, the 'failure' is never in eating a food below your stated trigger point or that the food itself is too fattening. It's the deeply unsatisfying experience of pacifying an urgent craving with an unworthy offering.

Be Demanding And Don't Settle For Good Enough.

Bad tasting foods are incompatible with a higher quality of life. Even mediocre-tasting foods are inconsistent with an enhanced sense of well-being. You must demand higher-quality foods for yourself. Insist on them.

A Jewish grandmother and her grandson are at the beach. He's playing in the water while she's standing on the shore not wanting to get her feet wet, when all of a sudden a huge wave appears from nowhere and crashes directly onto the spot where the boy is wading. The water recedes and the boy is no longer there. He was swept away.

The grandmother holds her hands to the sky, screams and cries: "Lord, how could you? Haven't I been a wonderful grandmother? Haven't I been a wonderful mother? Haven't I kept a kosher home? Haven't I given to the B'nai B'rith? Haven't I lit candles every Friday night? Haven't I tried my very best to live a life that you would be proud of?"

A voice booms from the sky: "All right already!"

A few minutes later another huge wave appears out of nowhere and crashes on the beach. As the water recedes, the boy is standing there. He is smiling and splashing around as if nothing had ever happened.

The voice booms again. "I have returned your grand-son. Are you satisfied?"

The grandmother says, *"He had a hat."*

Be demanding. Do not eat the bad-tasting just because it's healthy. Do not eat the mediocre-tasting just because it's there. Eat the delicious because it's the fastest way of achieving our well-being goal.

Maturing Taste Buds Means Smaller Waists.

A curious thing happens after spending a fair amount of time *Bargaining For Higher Quality Crap.* You start eating a whole lot less crap, whether it's high-quality or not. For example, I started eating less and less fast food because it just didn't taste as good as it once did. Big Macs are great, until you have a char-grilled burger from a better class of restaurant. Then suddenly the Big Mac just tastes salty. Today, it is rare for me to go to a fast food restaurant and it's a direct result of holding myself to a higher standard of crap. If I'm going to eat unhealthy I am going to eat DELI-CIOUS unhealthy, dammit.

This mentality had the salutary effect of cutting the volume and frequency of the low quality rubbish I was dining on. As your palate grows in sophistication your tolerance level for foods that could scare the moss off a rock decreases.

As my taste buds matured I stayed away from a lot of foods I once loved. Like Oreos. I rarely eat them anymore. How's that for irony? It wasn't a conscious decision. Over time, I kept choosing the highest-quality cookies, which made the Oreos seem rather mediocre. And that's how I naturally stopped or cut back on eating so many other fattening foods —not because I was on a diet, but because my sense of well-being guided me to better tasting foods.

How Can You Possibly Lose Weight with A System That Merely Postpones The Eating Of Fattening Foods?

It's a fair question and something that I often asked myself when I first started on this journey. There were times when my craving intensity for problem foods hit a "7" or above many times in a row. That meant I was eating a lot of burgers, fries and pizza.

There were times when I was surrounded by high-quality crap for weeks at a time (notably during holidays). That meant I was eating a lot of cookies, cakes and pies.

In those circumstances, I thought, how in the world can *Bargaining For Higher Quality Crap* or *Postponement Of The Goods* for that matter, do anything but accelerate weight gain? My inner dieter didn't understand how I could possibly lose weight with a delayed gratification strategy that merely postponed the inevitable.

I had all those fears and thoughts but they pretty much went away when I reminded myself that I wasn't on a diet—which I was on a journey to well-being, which *will result in weight loss.*

Once you get that mantra—and I mean *really* get it—your fears of gaining weight will melt away. You will ask yourself, as I did, a common sense question: "Why am I using short-term results to measure a long-term strategy?" It's like expecting to double your money with a retirement account that's three weeks old. Or expecting the value of a real estate purchase to appreciate a month after you bought it. Or expecting the launch of a new business to make money right away.

Make no mistake; delayed gratification is a long-term strategy. Both *Bargaining For Higher Quality Crap and Postponement Of The Goods* will help you lose weight <u>over time</u>. Yes, there will be times that you'll go on a run of "7" or higher cravings or that you'll be surrounded by high-quality crap on a constant basis but so what? If you're in that situation, remember three things:

1. Cravings tend to fluctuate wildly. Sometimes you go through a phase where they're relatively calm and other times when they're extreme. But over the long haul—months, a year or more—they even out. I've had cravings for fried chicken that were so high I ate it two or three times a week. They've also been so low that I've only eaten it once every two months. I kept my word through phases of high and low intensity cravings and I've been rewarded handsomely for it. Before I started on this path, do you know how many times I'd eaten potato chips when my craving for them were at a "2" or "3"? LOTS. Now I only eat them when the craving is a "7" or more. That's a huge decrease in potato chip consumption. And that's how *Postponing The Goods* helps you shed the pounds—you completely cut out low-craving indulgences.

"But, Michael," I hear you saying, "my cravings are always near a '10.' If I follow your advice I'm going to blow up like a balloon." If you go for more than a month or so with wildly strong cravings that are unmanageable you might, *might*, have an eating disorder like bulimia. I would definitely talk to your doctor or find out more about the subject by Googling "eating disorders." It is normal to have extended high-rank cravings that seem unmanageable for short periods of time, but if they never end you might be dealing with something best left to eating disorder specialists.

Assuming that you don't have an eating disorder, the question remains—how do you manage high-rank cravings for problem foods that go on for weeks at a time? Your first and best option is to do what I did —nothing. You go with the flow knowing that you are temporarily stuck in a short-term phase of a long-term journey. Your second option is to use the systematic desensitization process so that at least you're cutting the portions of problem foods.

2. You'll rarely be surrounded with high quality fat bombs. Unless you work in the food industry (restaurants, bakeries) it is rare to be constantly surrounded by high-quality crap. The opposite is true—we are virtually surrounded by low-quality garbage. You can't swing a cat without hitting a grocery store, a mini-mart, a gas station, a fast food joint, hell, even a high school hallway that isn't loaded with crappy, nutrition-free junk food. Trust me, your problem isn't going to be running from high-quality junk food; it's going to be finding it.

If you have high-intensity cravings and work in the hospitality industry or have a foodie family or do a lot of business entertaining where high-quality crap abounds, *Bargaining For Higher Quality Crap* will be harder but not terribly so. Just modify the bargaining to *Highest Quality Crap* (as opposed to *Higher Quality Crap*). Just because you're surrounded by foods with a higher quality list of ingredients than average doesn't necessarily mean they're all of equal quality, so go for the absolute highest. And remember, it isn't just about the quality of the ingredients but the taste of the food. I've eaten plenty of foods with top notch ingredients that tasted like the business end of a donkey.

3. You have an obligation to make healthy foods a priority. Delayed gratification techniques are critical to your success but they're far from the only ways we are going to meet our goals. As covered in Chapter Three, you are not absolved from the obligation to pursue healthy foods. Not because it will help you lose weight (although it will) but because a strong, healthy body supports your well-being. This is a BIG part of the overall plan. The delayed gratification tactics are simply there to control the consumption of problem foods. Reducing the volume and frequency of bad foods is healthy for you but not nearly as much as getting yourself to eat healthier options. It's not an either/or proposition. It's not about sacrificing problem foods for healthier options; it's about managing the intake of <u>all</u> foods in a mindful manner. If you find yourself in a high-intensity crave-fest the answer isn't to ditch the delayed gratification framework; it's to let it run its course while maximizing the consumption of the "Nutrilicious."

The Loss That Dare Not Speak Its Name.

Although weight loss is not our goal it would be naïve to pretend it isn't important. Whether you are two weeks away from being fat or two years into it, it's natural to obsess over weight loss. I acknowledge how hard it is to consider eating any food during the early stages of this process without thinking about its impact on your weight.

When I first started down this road I would look at the fried chicken on my plate and think, "How the hell is eating this going to help me lose weight?" Conversely, I would look at a "Nutrilicious" food, like my broccoli salad, and think, "Oooh, I'm glad I'm eating this because it will help me lose weight." If I was at the grocery store and couldn't decide whether I should buy a food or not I inevitably judged it on the basis of how well or how badly it would fare on my waistline.

We are all so used to checking the calorie, carbs, protein, sugar and fat contents in our food that we automatically judge them as either being good or bad for our BMI. It's so ingrained in us and we do it so compulsively that it would be naïve for me to suggest that you shouldn't do it. First, you do it automatically so it's not like you have a choice. But while you don't have the choice of thinking how a particular food is going to affect your weight you do have the choice of adding a thought right behind it. Namely, "Will eating this food add or subtract from my well-being?"

I submit to you that eating a plate of fried chicken adds to your well-being. I submit to you that eating organic salads add to your well-being. I submit to you that eating delicious foods, whether they are healthy or not, adds to your well-being.

We are using systematic desensitization and delayed gratification techniques to reduce the "bad but delicious" foods and the pursuit of healthier options to increase the good and luscious foods. TOGETHER, this strategy achieves our goal of well-being, which results in weight loss.

You Are Not On A Diet.

Eating "bad but delicious" foods like fried chicken does not represent weakness. It is not a sop we throw to the heathen within. It is not something we put up with for the greater good. It is *essential* to the greater good. We celebrate it as part of our master plan for well-being. If you are concerned that indulging in your highly-craved foods will make you gain weight it's only because you're not seeing the bigger picture.

You're also operating under the misguided notion that your body responds favorably to direct methods of losing weight. It doesn't. Science has proven over and over again that it's almost impossible to keep the weight off with direct approaches like traditional dieting.

Losing weight is not a simple affair. There are psychological, emotional, environmental, economic and physiological obstacles that keep you from reaching your goal in the same way that snow, ice, altitude sickness, avalanches, faulty equipment, and crevasses are obstacles that can keep you from reaching the top of the mountain.

Weight loss is not a gentle sloping hill that you can climb with flip-flops in a matter of hours. It's more like Annapurna, the world's deadliest peak. You can't do it in flip-flops. It's going to take you months. You're going to need a whole lot of equipment, a whole lot of training and a good lawyer to help you write a will.

It's worth remembering that as you bargain for higher quality, better-tasting crap, you will eliminate the lower quality, bad tasting stuff. Lower quality crap is everywhere and you are going to slowly eliminate it from your diet. Higher-quality crap is harder to come by and you are going to add it. Now do the math: if you eliminate a lot and add a little what does that leave you with? Weight loss.

But it is weight loss over time. Lots of time. Not days or weeks but months and months. But they are months and months of enjoyable eating. Months and months of increasing well-being. Months and months of laying the foundation to a happier life—a life of having mouthwatering foods you love without worrying about your weight.

Sounds like a pretty good deal to me.

Where Are We?

We shifted our goal from weight loss to well-being. We are not on a diet; we are on a journey to well-being, which results in weight loss.

We avoid triggering the body's fat-promoting biological responses to dieting. We don't restrict or ban foods, set weight loss goals, or weigh ourselves constantly.

We use pain-free systematic desensitization techniques to reduce or eliminate binging. The reduction of sugar and fat enhances our sense of well-being, which results in weight loss.

We are committed to eating healthy foods. We go for the "Nutrilicious"—healthy foods that are delicious to you, even if they're mixed with not-so-healthy ingredients.

We use two delayed gratification techniques, Postponement Of The Goods and Bargaining For Higher Quality Crap, to reduce the frequency with which we eat problem foods. We know that "No never means no. It means later."

CHAPTER SIX

How To End Low-Craving Eating
& Low-Quality Indulgences

*Combining Both Delayed Gratification Techniques
To Pack A Bigger Punch*

Postponing The Goods & *Bargaining For Higher Quality Crap* are both delayed gratification techniques that motivate you with the promise of a better eating experience. Fulfilling an intense craving is far more satisfying than fulfilling a weak one. And eating high quality crap is far more satisfying than eating low-quality junk. Eliminating or reducing low-craving eating and low-quality indulgences enhances your well-being, which results in weight loss. You get to eat what you like AND lose/maintain weight. Not a bad deal. But there is a better one to be had: Combining both delayed gratification techniques as they will result in greater pleasure, greater well-being and, dare I say it, greater weight loss.

I strongly suggest you don't try combining the two delayed gratification techniques until both have become such ingrained habits that, like brushing your teeth before bed, you do them without thinking (about 3-6 months). Let's review both delayed gratification techniques:

Postponing The Goods

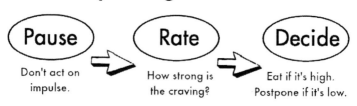

Pause — Don't act on impulse.

Rate — How strong is the craving?

Decide — Eat if it's high. Postpone if it's low.

Bargaining For Higher Quality Crap

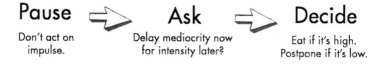

Pause — Don't act on impulse.

Ask — Delay mediocrity now for intensity later?

Decide — Eat if it's high. Postpone if it's low.

So how do I combine the two techniques? First, I rate my craving. If it hits my '7' trigger point I then ask if I'm willing to bargain for something better. So now food has to jump through two hoops before it lands in my stomach—high craving and high quality.

It took me a while to get the hang of it but today I don't care if my craving elevates to Defcon 5, I will not eat a food if it isn't of high quality. That may not make sense at first. I mean, why would I be craving for a terrible tasting food?

Well, you don't always know if a food's good until you taste it. Ever have a delicious looking apple that tasted like wax? Or a scrumptious looking cookie that tasted like spackle? Or crispy-looking fried chicken that tasted stale? I could go on. Once you get the basics of the *Postponing* & *Bargaining* delayed gratification techniques you'll be ready to make the deal I make for myself: Do not eat mediocre-tasting problem foods even if they have high-quality ingredients and your craving for it is sky-high.

It is a commitment I made to my well-being. I do not eat bland or mediocre foods that are unhealthy for me. I only eat delicious foods that are unhealthy for me! My rule is so strong that if I bite into a homemade, delicious-looking but bland-tasting cookie, I will spit it out mid-bite.

That may sound vaguely eating disordered to some, fanatically self-disciplined to others and incredibly rude to most (especially if I'm next to the person who baked it!) but to me it's simply what happens when you graduate to an advanced version of my delayed gratification techniques. When you train your body long enough with these techniques it automatically rejects bad or mediocre-tasting foods.

This is an evolutionary process. Again, I would not try combining the two delayed gratification techniques until you get the hang of them separately. And even then, you do not need to combine them to achieve your goals. Combining the two techniques is simply a more advanced option.

Postponing The Goods +
Bargaining For Higher Quality Crap

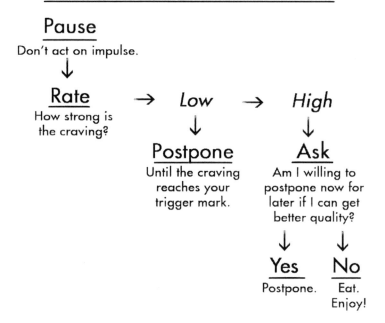

Pause
Don't act on impulse.

↓

Rate → *Low* → *High*
How strong is
the craving?

↓ ↓

Postpone ## Ask
Until the craving | Am I willing to
reaches your | postpone now for
trigger mark. | later if I can get
| better quality?

↓ ↓

Yes ## No
Postpone. | Eat.
| Enjoy!

Option or not, my philosophy still holds: I do not sacrifice my well-being (which includes health and weight considerations) on bad or mediocre-tasting fat bombs. For example, I had a box of Whole Foods gourmet crackers in the covert that I had never tried. I wanted it desperately. It was so 'bleh' I spit it out onto a napkin and held the box above the trashcan. Suddenly, I had an internal argument going on in my head. My inner cheapskate hissed, "Dammit, Michael, that box cost $18!" But my well-being advocate whispered, "Life's too short to eat food the dog would find questionable."

The box hit the trash can harder than the bottom of a whiskey bottle at an Irish wake.

I am willing to sacrifice my well-being for "good tasting bad food" if it's so tasty I'd sit up and bark for it. I am not, however, willing to do it for something that makes me roll over and play dead. Again, here's how combining the two delayed gratification techniques work:

- Your craving must meet your trigger point.

- It must have high-quality ingredients.

- It must taste delicious (high-quality ingredients are a signal of tastiness but not a guarantee).

This is a 3 out of 3 proposition. Not 1 of 3 or 2 of 3. All three elements must be present before I give myself the go-ahead. You will be surprised how easy this is to do once you experience "Food Nirvana" over and over again. Food Nirvana is that moment when desire, taste and high caliber contents come together so powerfully that it makes you incapable of thought. Once you experience it multiple times you'll want to keep replicating it and suddenly you'll have trained your body to want it so badly that it's willing to delay gratification for it.

Food Nirvana

Intense Craving + High Quality Ingredients
+ Delicious Taste

Food Nirvana is highly individual. What you may find tasty I might find grounds for arrest. I recommend that you constantly look for ways to eat what you like, not simply what is there.

Scenario

You want French fries but your friends decided on a restaurant that serves the crappy kind. You've eaten here before so you know, but even if you haven't you can see the fries on other diners' plates and they don't look all that appetizing.

Pause: Should you order them?

Rate: How badly do you want fries? Let's say it's a '9' craving.

Ask: Are you willing to delay a mediocre experience now if you guarantee you'll have a more intense one later?

Decide: No? Then eat. Mangia mangia! Yes? Then postpone but make sure you get to a place that serves great fries soon.

Discussion: The battle between a high craving and a low tolerance for crap is never easy. Early on I used to go ahead and eat the crappy fries because the craving over-powered me. But those indulgences also fortified my later decision-making because I remembered how dissatisfying it was to stoke a '9' craving for fries with a serving that tasted so bad it made me lose my short-term memory.

It's important that you <u>guarantee</u> the later pleasure. When I have an especially strong craving for fries but only question-able ones are available, I will say or think something like this: "I promise if I skip this mediocre crap I'll take myself to a place that makes fries so good I'll want to lick other people's fingers." Then I'll actually think back to places that serve great fries and make up my mind to go there next time.

The more detailed you make your postponement promise the easier it will be for you to delay. Don't say, "Sometime in the next couple of months I'll have excellent fries some-where." Say, "I'm going to Marlowe's Tavern on Tuesday and get a large portion of their fries."

Again, you don't have to do an advanced combination of *Postponing The Goods* and *Bargaining For Higher Quality Crap* to achieve your goals. They're perfectly fine as stand-alone techniques. Both are guided by mindfulness and both will enhance your well-being, which will eventually reduce the junk in your trunk.

CHAPTER SEVEN

Keep Everything You've Learned From Falling Off The Kitchen Table

A Review Of Important Concepts, Resources and Last Minute Tips

I see a bright, slim future for you. After all, you're only a few reframes away from a significantly better sense of well-being, and you know what that means: Weight loss!

That's the good news. The bad news is that you've been so conditioned to expect instant results ("Lose ten pounds by the end of the week!") that the pace of your progress might discourage you. Don't be. You can't undo in a couple of weeks what took years to build. If I had an instant tele-portation machine that would deposit you at the end of your journey, I'd give it to you, but I don't, so we're going to have to rely on taking a trip the old-fashioned way—by putting one foot in front of the other.

The journey begins by applying a 3-step process—*Reframe* your goals from weight loss to health enhancement, *Eliminate* binge eating through desensitization and *Reduce* the volume and frequency of problem food consumption through innovative delayed gratification techniques.

I can boil the results of the Scratch Plan down to one word: Moderation. It's the key to losing/maintaining weight without going on a diet. Moderation is essentially about volume control. Eat less volume lose more weight. Moderation is simple: Eat what you want but only if you really want it and in reasonable portions.

Moderation is an easy place to live; it's just damn hard getting there. If moderation is a fantastic penthouse with every conceivable amenity it's also 40 floors up with no apparent staircase or elevator. The techniques in this book function as an elevator that open directly into the penthouse living room. It's a slow ride up, but man, look at that view! And once you're up there, life is easy.

Slim, too.

The desensitization, habituation and delayed gratification techniques in the Scratch Plan are all about a painless ascension into the penthouse of moderation. You implement small but attainable reductions in your everyday eating habits and you achieve long-term behavioral changes and weight loss.

There is no such thing as a food you can't or shouldn't have in your journey to well-being. There is only how much and how frequently you can have them.

Get Thinner With Skinner.

I owe much of my Scratch Plan theories to B.F. Skinner (considered one of the most influential psychologists of the 20th century). Behavior modification is at the heart of desensitization, habituation, and delayed gratification. But the Scratch Plan is also mixed with mindfulness—the ability to tell the difference between habit and hunger and to distinguish between a slight desire and a stronger one. In a lot of ways The Scratch Plan is about behaving your way into new thinking and thinking your way into new behavior.

The result, as I said, is being able to eat moderately. And once you can do that the system is self-perpetuating. There are many studies documenting the power of smaller portions to "shrink" your stomach over time. Scientific evidence shows that once you start eating smaller portions your stomach stops asking for larger ones. I am Exhibit A of that phenomenon. Once I calmly reduced my intake of Oreos from 16 to 3 I never, EVER had a craving for that many cookies anymore.

How is it possible to be just as satisfied with 3 Oreos as I once was with 16? Because the body adapts easily to change *as long as the change comes in small, almost imperceptible increments.* You simply condition your body to become full after consuming a smaller quantity of food. Eating moderate portions rather than overly large ones will also make you feel better (it improves the digestive process) and gives you more energy.

Remember, you don't need a food plan to lose weight; you need an eating strategy. Moderation doesn't mean eating tiny portions of whatever you want but leaving the table hungry. It means eating whatever you want but reducing the amount of food needed to make you feel full.

Before I go over the 7 major concepts in this book I'd like to share a couple of resources you'll find enormously helpful:

The Marshmallow Test, by Walter Mischel.
This is easily the best, most interesting book on self-control I've ever read.

The Power of Habit, by Charles Duhigg.
A worthy addition to the habit-forming shelf in your library.

Switch: How to Change Things When Change Is Hard, by Chip Heath
A great tome on making everlasting changes.

Mindless Eating, by Brian Wansink.
A profound book that had a huge impact on me.

The Food Lab, at Cornell University
Simply the most compelling food research studies on the Internet. http://foodpsychology.cornell.edu/

Some Things Are Worth Going Over Again.

True story. A missionary friend worried about the high pregnancy rate in a Kenyan village tried an experiment with condoms. To start, she chose this one African woman who kept getting pregnant. My friend tells her about condoms. The woman stares blankly. My friend shows her how to use it by unrolling it over a broomstick. "Ahh!" The woman brightens up. A few months later the woman's pregnant again. My friend says "Didn't you use the condoms?" The woman says "Yes. Every day I unrolled it over the broomstick before we made love."

My point, and I do have one, is that sometimes understanding new concepts demands repetition. So, in case you're still looking for a broomstick I'd like to repeat the central tenets of this book:

1. **Dieting Doesn't Work.**
   Dieting creates fat-promoting biological responses (it slows your metabolism and makes you hungrier). The only way to avoid the boomerang effect of deprivation is to stop dieting.

2. **You Can Lose Weight Without Dieting.**
   How? By aiming for a higher goal whose attainment *results* in weight loss. That goal is a peak sense of well-being, a higher quality of life, which requires you to eat healthy meals and take great pleasure out of food. These two goals (healthy foods and pleasure)

are often at odds with each other. Therefore you must eat healthy AND indulge in not-so-healthy foods. You cannot achieve a sense of well-being by being healthy but unhappy with what you're eating.

3. Change Will Come Slowly.

The only way you can lose weight without sending your body into Defcon 5 mode is to make slow, gradual, almost imperceptible changes. You can achieve instant results with a diet but they're temporary. You can achieve permanent results with the Scratch Plan but they're gradual. Choose permanence over immediacy.

4. Eat Healthier By Moving Toward The Nutrilicious.

You can eat healthier (and enjoy it) by aiming for the "Nutrilicious"—a nutritionally dense vegetable, fruit or fish mixed with not-as-healthy foods to make it appealing *to you*. It's a fusion between healthy-but-boring foods and unhealthy-but-exciting. Remember, the best healthy foods are the ones you'll eat. For that, you need a compass not a map. You are aiming for direction, not perfection.

5. Use Desensitization And Habituation To Stop Binging.

The point isn't to deprive yourself of pleasurable

foods, it's to eat them in moderate portions. Remember, an enhanced sense of well-being *requires* you to eat yummy comfort food even if they're not healthy for you.

6. Use The Pleasure Principle To Reduce Intake Of "Bad" Foods.

The point isn't to "cut down." That's diet-speak. The point is to only eat high calorie foods when your craving for them is sky high. Remember, a plate of spaghetti and meatballs (with garlic bread!) will taste a lot better when your craving for it hits a "10" than when it's a "2." Doing this will almost completely eliminate low-craving eating, which some scientists think makes up to 25% of our caloric intake. *Postponing The Goods* is a delayed gratification technique that will help you do that.

The premise behind *Postponement Of The Goods*: You are not going to deny yourself a problem meal; you're going to postpone its consumption to a later date when your craving for it is at a higher level. Your options are not "eat" or "don't eat." They're "eat" or "postpone." No never means no. It means later. No means you're on a diet. Later means you're waiting for a better time to enjoy the food. You can cut out a third to two thirds of your problem foods not by deprivation but by postponement.

7. Use The Pleasure Principle To "Trade Up."

Mediocre-tasting foods are inconsistent with an enhanced sense of well-being. You must demand higher-quality foods for yourself. The higher the quality the more pleasure you will get out of food, which consequently enhances your well-being. So set a higher threshold for quality. You can do that with a delayed gratification technique I call, *Bargaining for Higher Quality Crap.* When you replace low-quality ingredients (say, packaged cookies out of a vending machine) with high-quality ingredients (Aunt Edna's homemade chocolate chip cookies) you not only will get more pleasure out of it, you will improve your health.

> The main premise behind *Bargaining For Higher Quality Crap*: Say no to crap now so you can have higher-quality crap later. Don't deny yourself foods you crave; postpone eating them until you can find a higher quality version. The question is simple. "Am I willing to postpone eating this today for something better tomorrow?"

These are the seven major concepts in the book. Understand them well as they will serve you well. Now, I want to share some tidbits to tide you over some of the more challenging moments you may have on the road to enhanced well-being.

Can I Have Some More?

It's not about sacrificing problem foods for healthier options; it's about managing the intake of <u>all</u> foods in a mindful manner.

Let's talk about cravings in a context I have not previously mentioned: Second helpings. How do you handle them? What if the cravings are strong? You already know the answer to that: If it hits a pre-agreed trigger (like a "7") then go for it. But sometimes your cravings are heavily influenced by environmental factors like watching those around you reach for seconds or internal factors like your emotional state. Is there any way to take these factors into account?

Yes. Call a time out. Postpone the decision to eat for 90 seconds. Look at your watch and say to yourself, "In 90 seconds I will rate my craving for that second piece of cake. And if it's still banging at a '7' or more I will eat it with pleasure."

Don't stare at your watch for the duration of your "time-out." Engage with other people or if you're alone, pet the dog or feed the cat. Don't let the urgency of a craving throw you into immediacy. You're not on a diet but you are on a journey toward well-being. Food impulsivity rarely enhances well-being. Mindfulness does. Make your decision when the clock runs out. You'll be amazed at how a minute and half can lower the craving by a couple of points—enough for you to delay consumption to the near future with mild disappointment rather than intolerable pain.

Take Smaller Mouthfuls

A funny thing happened to me on the way toward ending my binges on Oreos. I learned that you can use desensitization and habituation in the most unusual ways. For instance, I noticed that I tended to use my eating utensils as shovels rather than forks, knives and spoons. It takes your stomach about 20 minutes to fully recognize satiety so it stands to reason that the slower you eat the better you'll be at recognizing when you're full. At first, I dramatically reduced the amount of food I'd fork. You can imagine how well that worked out. *Immensely dissatisfying.* But then I remembered the principles of desensitization and slowly, gradually, almost imperceptibly, reduced the amount of food I'd spear onto my fork. It worked!

I encourage you to look at any aspect of your eating and see where you can apply desensitization and habituation to it.

Put It In Smaller Bowls & Plates.

One of the best ways to maintain moderation—once you achieve it through desensitization, habituation and delayed gratification—is to capitalize on a visual perception bias called the Delboeuf Illusion.

The Delboeuf Illusion states that surroundings affect perceptions of size. The same amount of food sitting on a big plate is going to seem much smaller than if it's sitting on a small one. The reverse is true. The same amount of food sitting on a small plate is going to seem much bigger than if it were on a big plate.

Why does this matter? Because you will feel fuller after eating from the smaller plate than if you eat from the larger one, even though it's the same amount of food. How's that for straight-jacket crazy?

Picture two scenarios:

> **Scenario #1:** Your host serves you 8 oz of hearty soup in a 16-oz bowl. The soup fills half the bowl. You look at it and think, "What a stingy host!"

> **Scenario #2:** Your host serves you 8 oz of hearty soup in a 9-oz bowl. The soup looks like it might spill onto the table. You think, "What a generous host!"

Study after study at Cornell University's Food Lab shows that you will feel far more satiated after eating the 8 oz of soup if it's served in the smaller bowl. Why? The Delboeuf Illusion makes you think you've eaten more food. The illusion is so strong that even when subjects eating out of smaller bowls were told of the illusion they still reported stronger feelings of satiation.

The Delboeuf Illusion also applies to serving bowls. The bigger the bowl, the more food you'll take. The smaller the bowl, the less you'll take. And guess what? You'll feel just as full in either case. One study found that 77% more pasta was taken and 71% more was consumed when people served themselves from the large bowl as compared to a medium bowl.

Bottom line? Serve yourself from medium bowls and put the food in smaller bowls. You'll feel just as satisfied and not even notice that you've eaten a lot less food.

Buy Smaller Dishes

According to experts, the average size of an American dinner plate has increased almost 23% since 1900. This argues for restocking your pantry with smaller dishes, or at the very least, using the smallest dishes in your collection.

Buy Taller Glasses.

The Delboeuf Illusion also affects your drinking habits. When asked to pour equal amounts of a liquid into a short, wide glass and a tall, skinny one, studies show that even experienced bartenders poured too much into the short, wide glass. That's because we tend to overestimate vertical lengths and underestimate horizontal lengths.

This finding has obvious implications for anything that you drink too much of. Want a milkshake? Pour it into a tall, thin glass. You'll pour less, drink less and be just as satisfied as if you'd had more. The same goes for alcohol. If you want to cut down, or at least slow down, pour your nectar into tall and thin stemware.

Gratify Your Oral Needs

Do you really have a craving for that candy bar or does your mouth simply need to be stimulated? Everybody has an oral fixation of some kind. You can really see it in smokers. It's not just about the nicotine—it's about having something in their mouths. Many a quitter has discovered that the stimulation of chewing (usually gum) is one of the best ways to manage their oral fixation.

Try chewing sugar-free gum or sucking on a hard candy. Or if you really want to get adventurous, eat a fruit like an apricot or a peach, then suck on the pits for the next half hour. The point isn't to avoid the food you're craving (that would be a diet and we're not on one). The point is to distinguish between a real craving and the need for oral stimulation.

Don't Get Blinded By Diets.

Finally, I'd like to share an interesting tale from a Sufi philosopher:

A man was walking past the home of the Sufi rascal-sage Nasrudin one evening when he saw Nasrudin on his hands and knees searching for something under a streetlight. "Did you lose something?" asked the passerby.

"My house keys," answered Nasrudin, distraught.

Being a good Samaritan, the man got down on his knees and began patting the grass along with Nasrudin.

A few minutes later another neighbor came by and joined in the search. Then another friend, and another, until a whole group of people were scouring the area.

After a long search, no one had any success. Finally someone asked Nasrudin, "Do you remember where you were standing when you dropped your keys?"

"Yes," answered Nasrudin. "I was standing over there," he explained, pointing to a darkened area quite far from where everyone was searching. "Then why are you looking over here?" asked one of his helpers.

"It was easier to look under the streetlight," answered Nasrudin.

Most of us search for the keys to weight loss under the bright lights of a diet. We toil endlessly without reward simply because we don't know where else to look. I hope I illuminated the darkened areas enough so that you could point to the keys and say, "Oh, look! There they are!"

Other Books by Michael Alvear

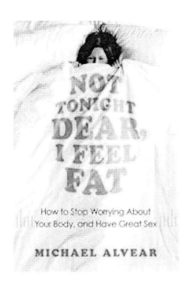

Read this remarkable guide and find out how to:

- Shut off the negative thoughts about your body before, during and after sex.

- Use sex techniques that will make you forget to "check" your thighs or worry about your partner seeing something you're ashamed of.

- Stop panicking when your partner touches a body part you're self-conscious about.

Available at bookstores everywhere.

CPSIA information can be obtained at www.ICGtesting.com
Printed in the USA
LVOW11s1729171115

462996LV00001B/16/P